INTERMITTENT

FASTING

FOR WOMEN OVER 40

cherish yourself again with proven recipes to lose weight, reset metabolism and enhance energy | 28 days meal plan included

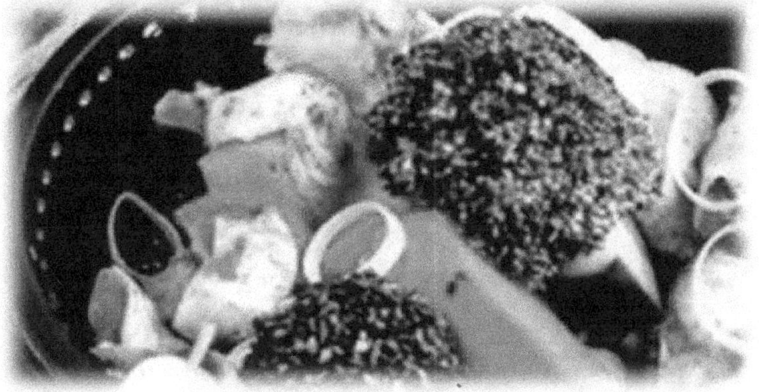

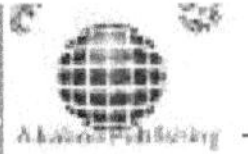

Dr. Grace Hester Alkalosis Publishing

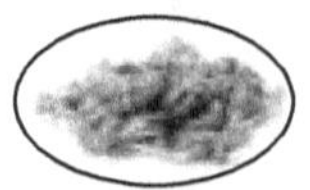 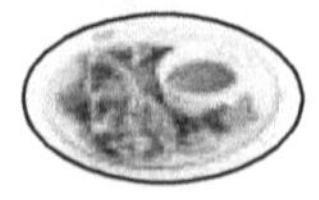 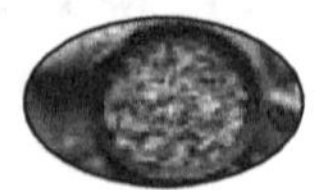

Copyright Page

DR. GRACE HESTER

Dr. Grace Hester stands at the intersection of health, passion, and culinary excellence. A distinguished medical professional and accomplished nutritionist, she seamlessly weaves together her expertise to create a holistic approach to well-being.

Dr. Hester earned her medical degree from the renowned Johns Hopkins School of Medicine, consistently ranked among the top medical schools globally. Her commitment to advancing healthcare led her to prestigious positions at the Mayo Clinic, where she honed her skills in internal medicine. Driven by a desire to explore the profound connection between nutrition and overall health, she furthered her education at the Culinary Institute of America.

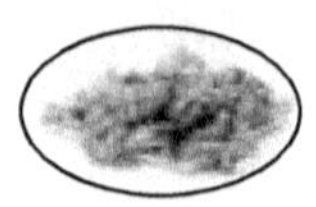 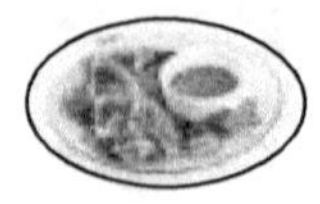 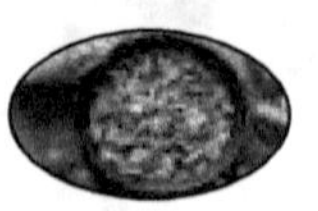

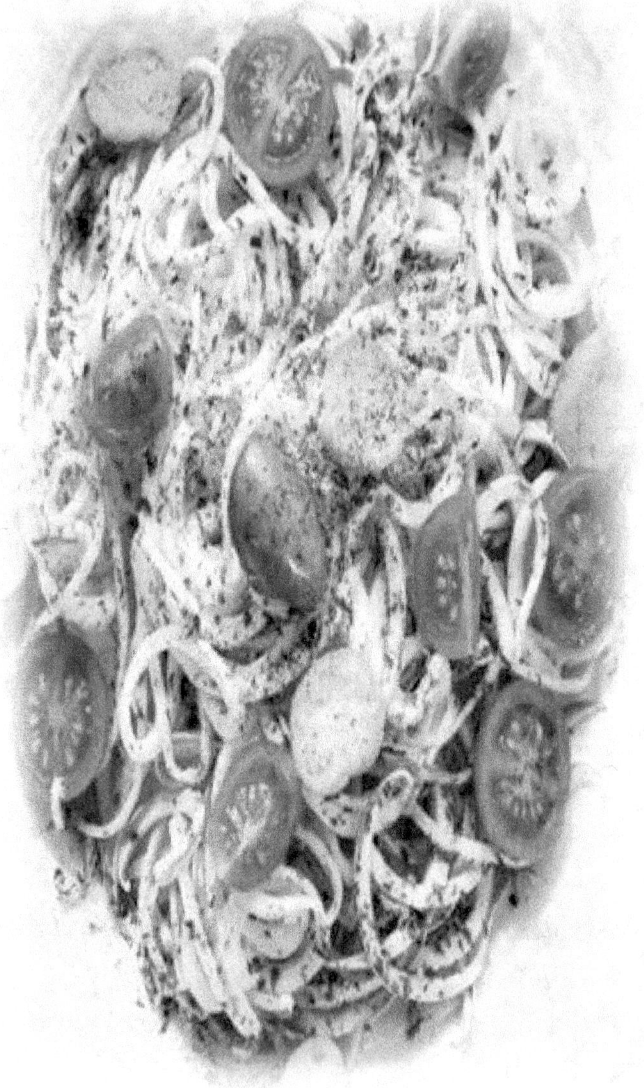

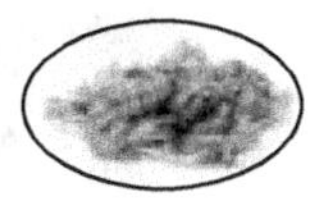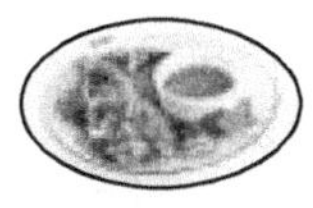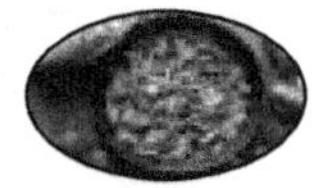

TABLE OF CONTENT–

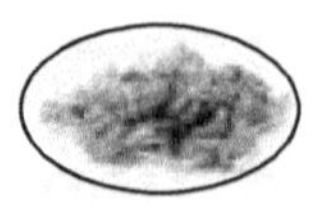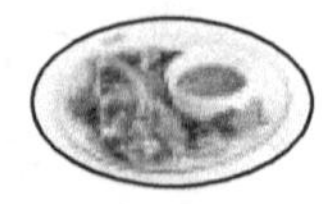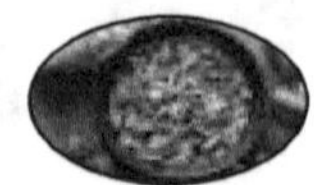

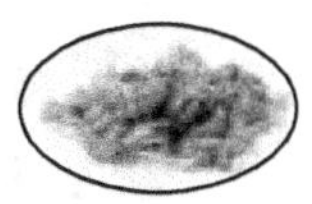 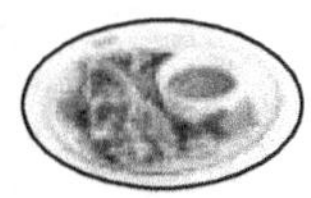 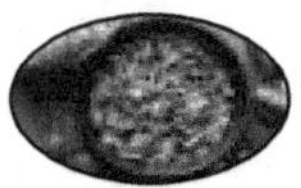

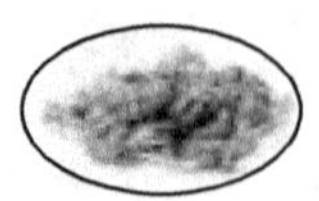 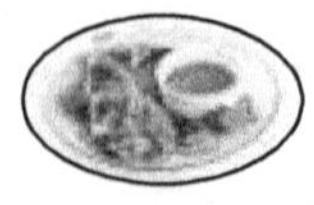 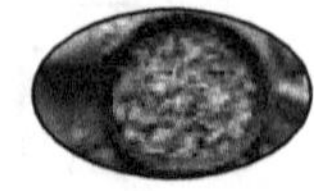

28-DAY INTERMITTENT FASTING MEAL PLAN

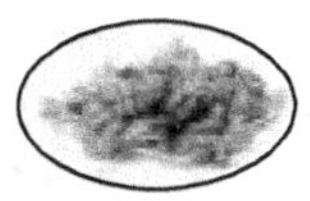 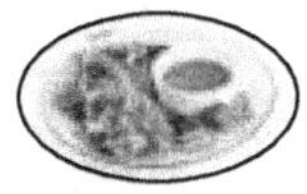 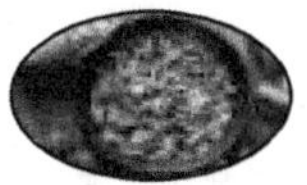

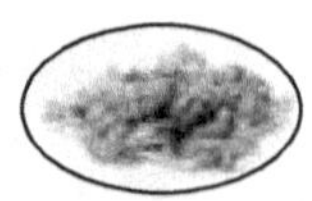 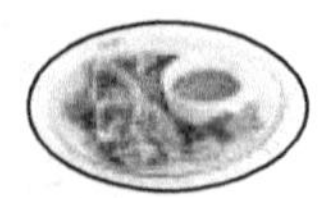 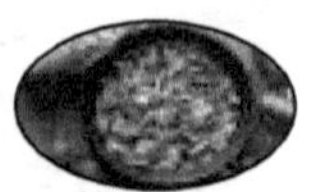

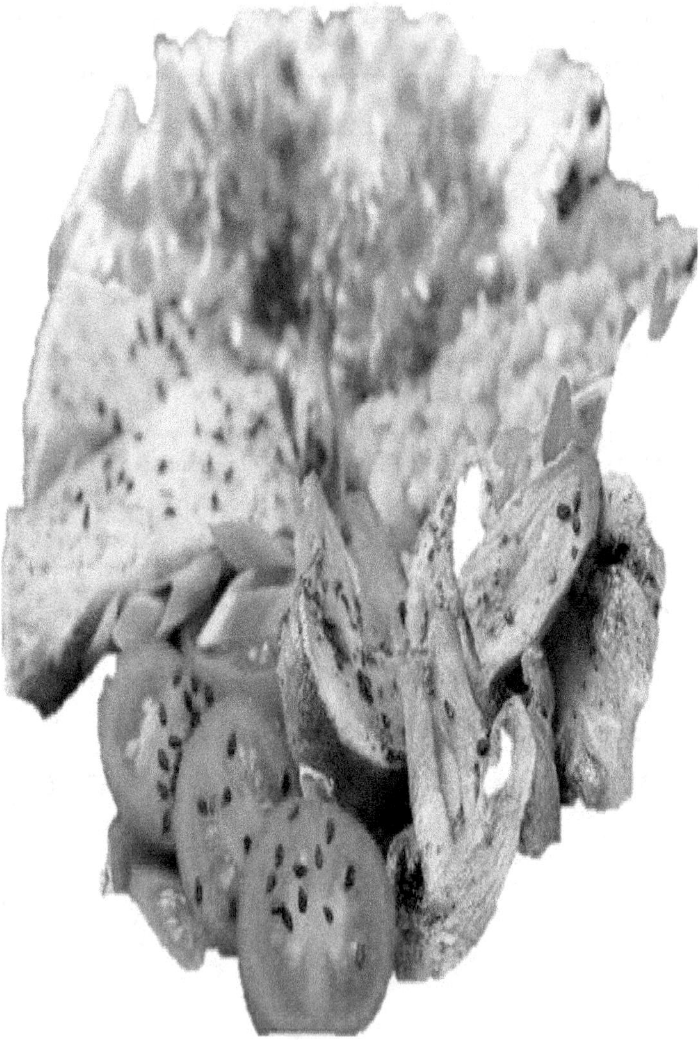

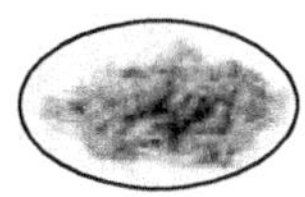 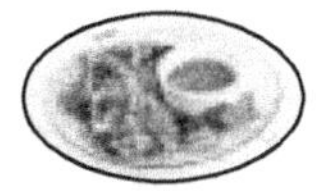 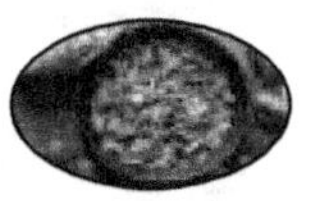

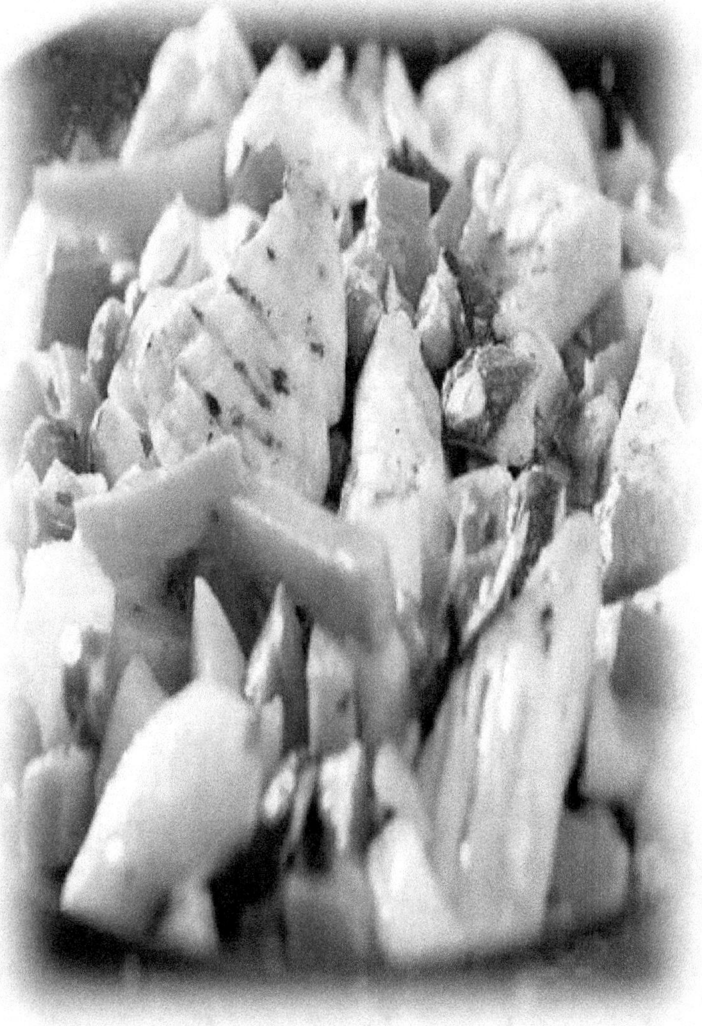

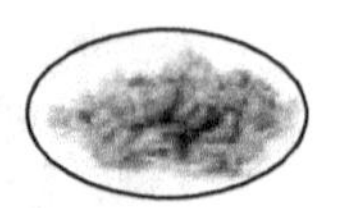
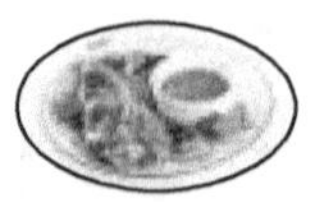
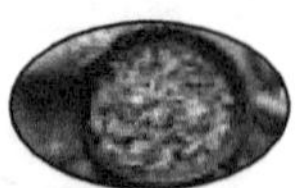
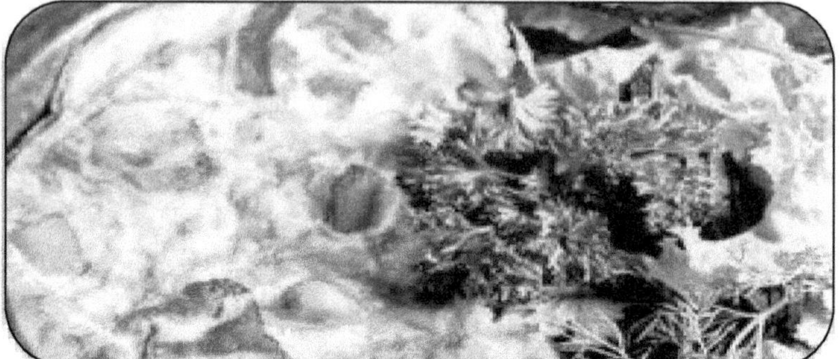
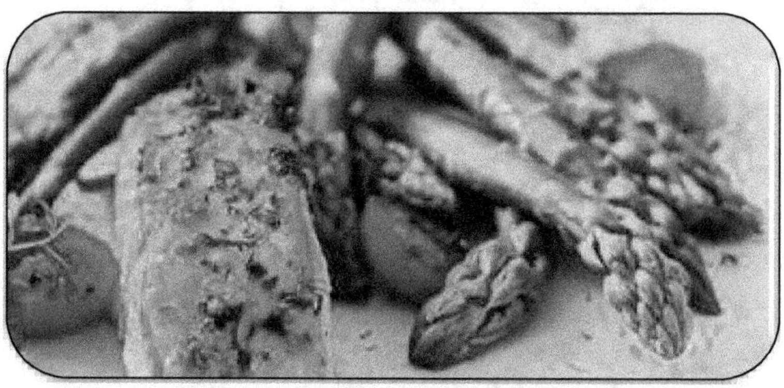
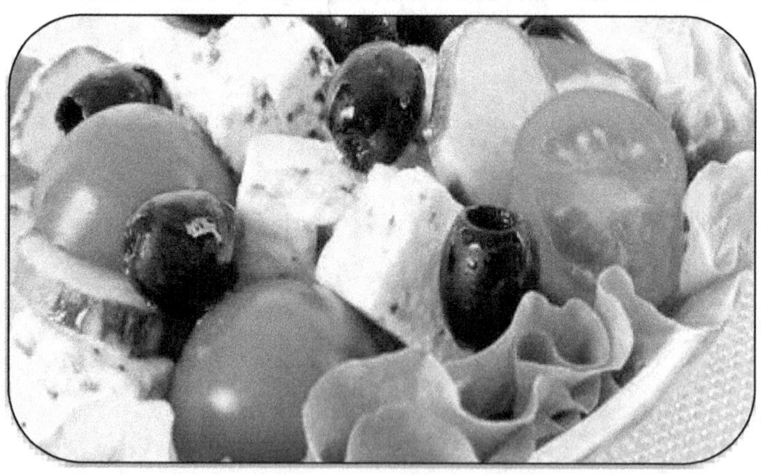

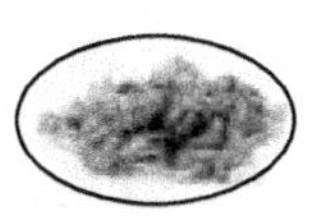 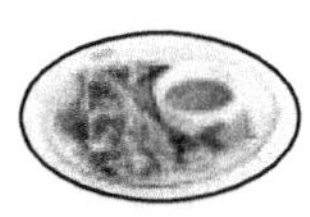 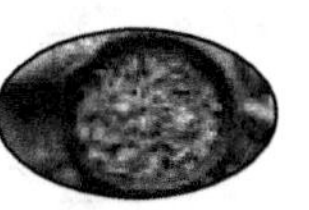

Diet

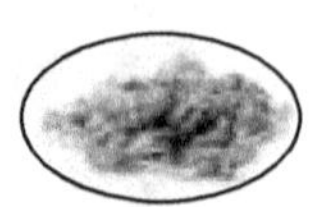 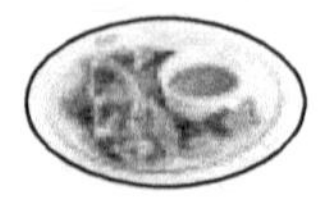 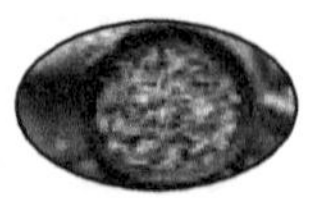

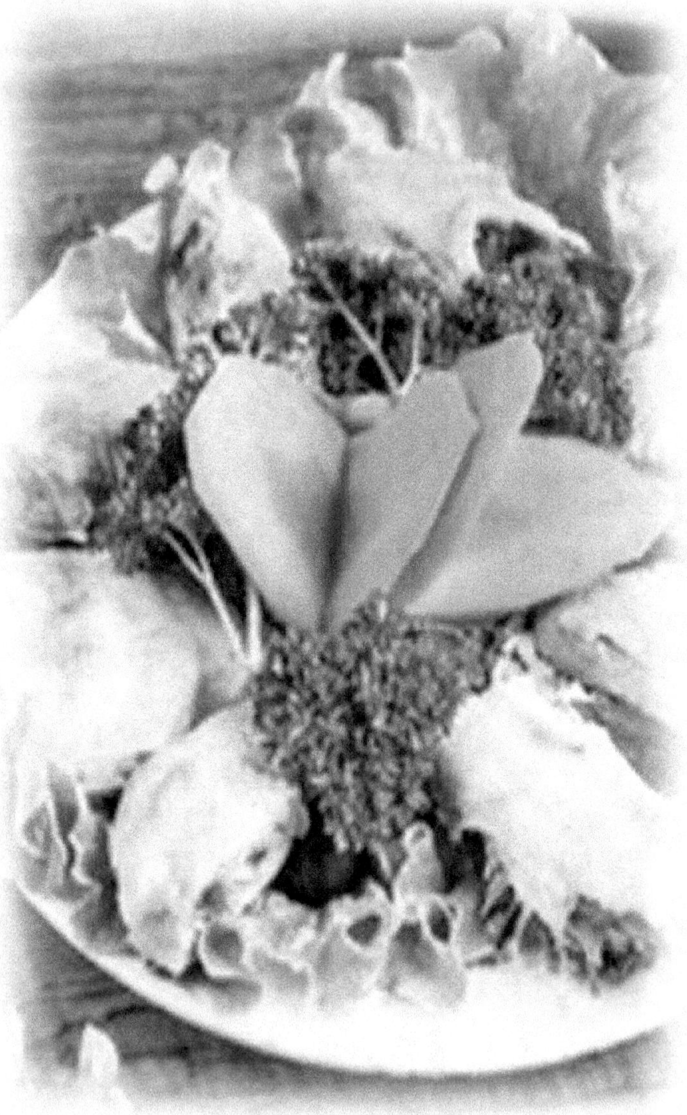

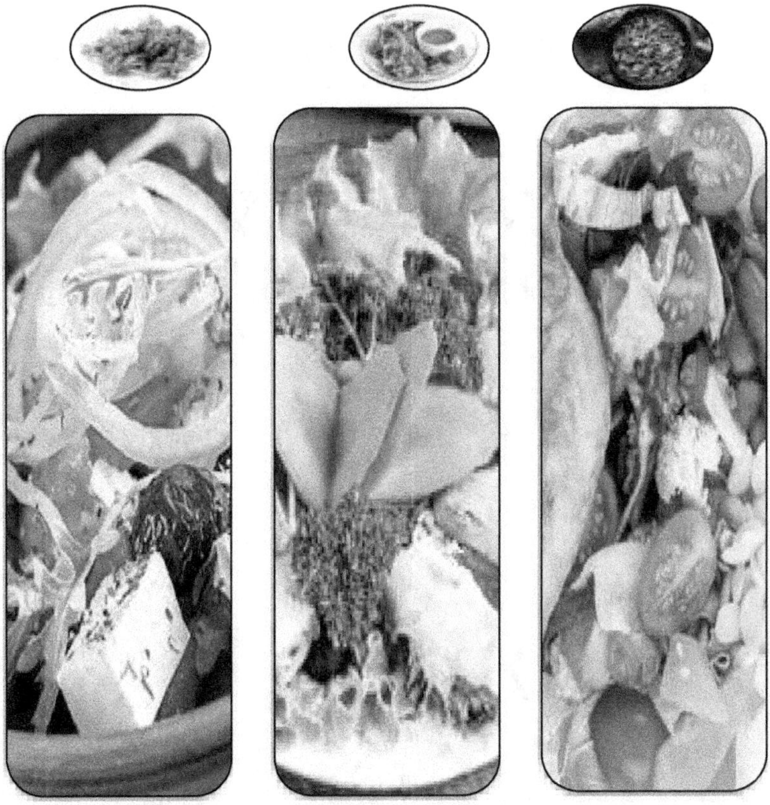

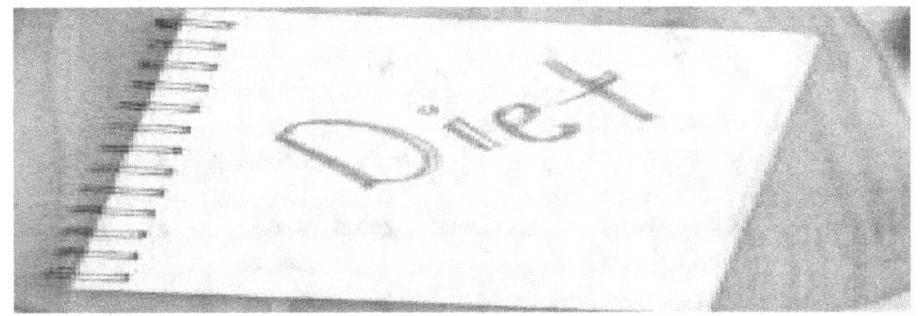
Diet

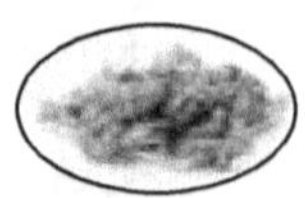 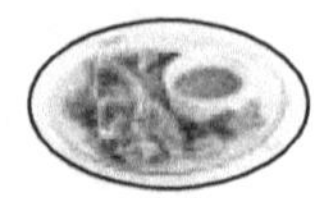 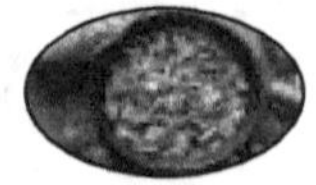

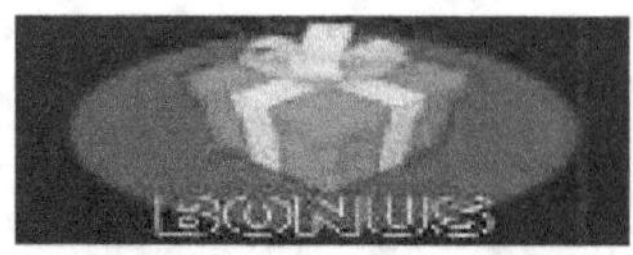

SCAN THE QR CODE TO GET YOUR FREE HOME MADE GREEN SMOOTHIE RECIPE BOOK

BONUS 1

Your 20 days meal planner is attached at the end of the book. Enjoy!

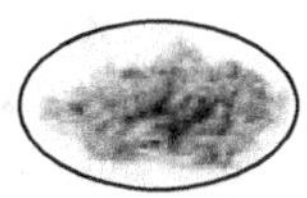 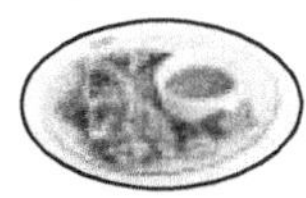 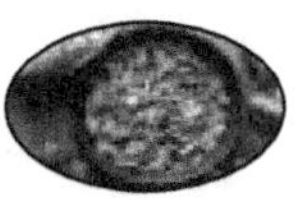

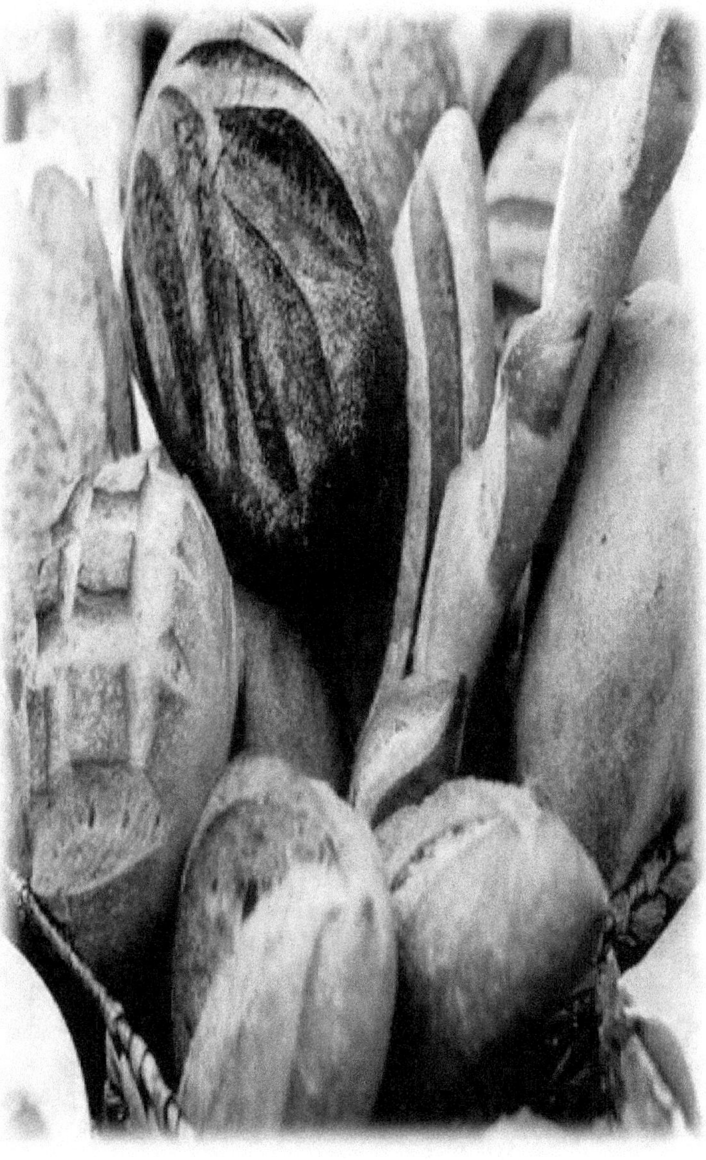

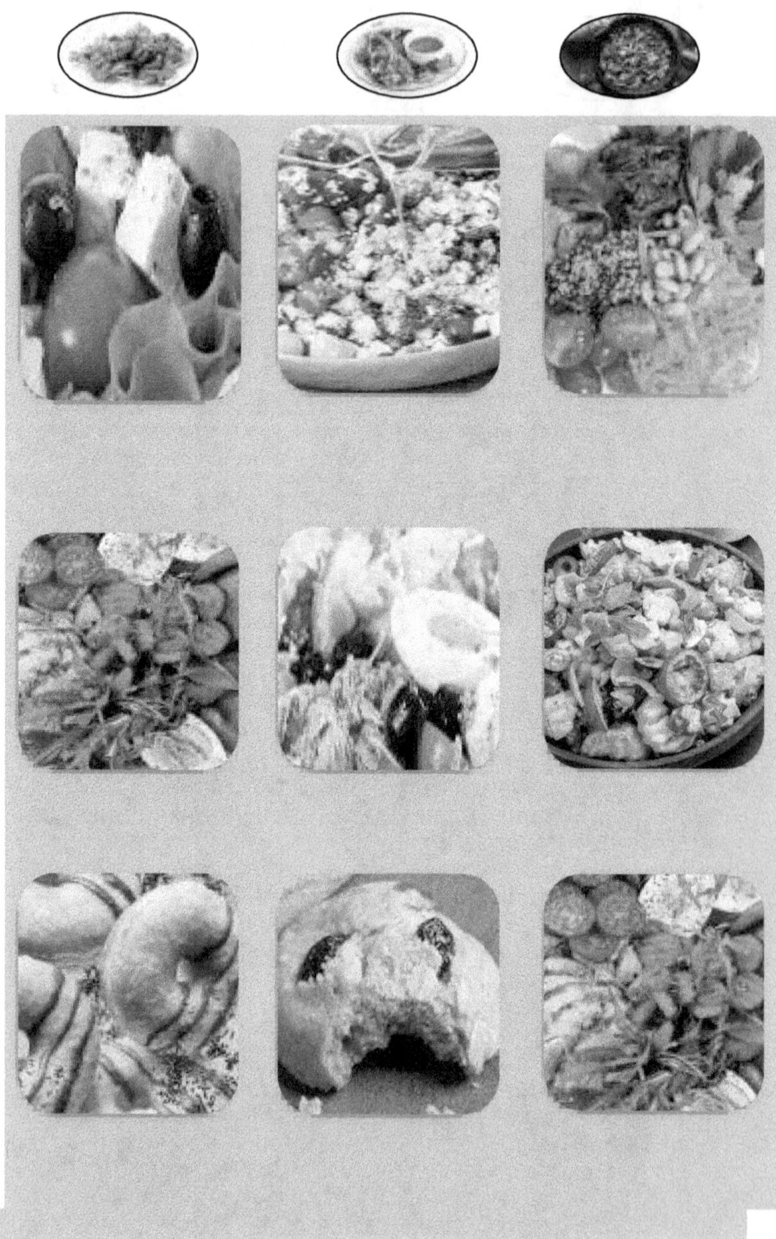

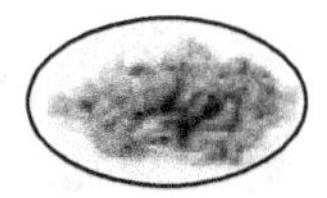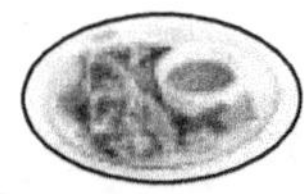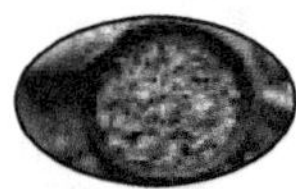

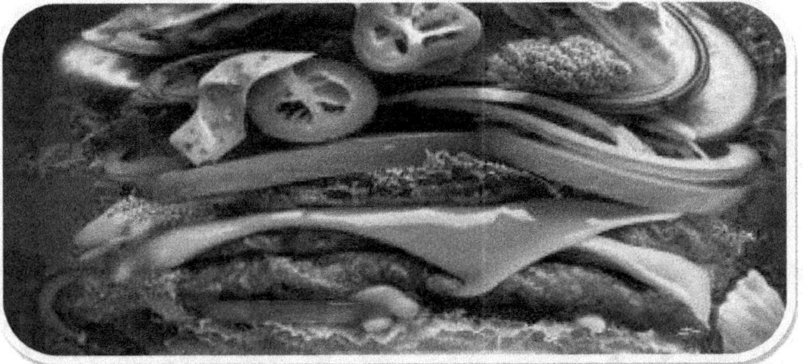

INTRODUCTION–

In the quiet town of Harmonyville, where time seemed to slow down and the community held a tight bond, lived a remarkable woman named Emily. At the age of 52, Emily found herself at a crossroads. Despite her best efforts to maintain a healthy lifestyle, the pounds had slowly crept up on her, and a sense of fatigue seemed to have settled in.

One day, while chatting with her lifelong friend Sarah during their weekly walking session, Emily discovered the transformative power of intermittent fasting. Sarah, a vibrant 55-year-old, spoke animatedly about how this approach had –

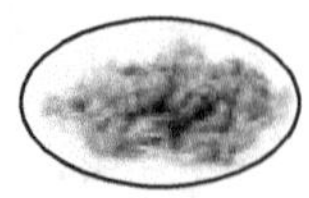 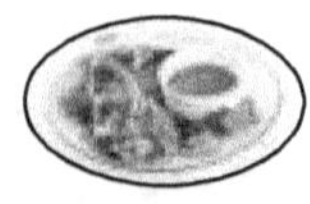 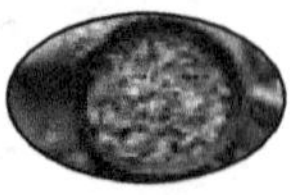

not only helped her shed unwanted weight but had also revitalized her energy and mental clarity.

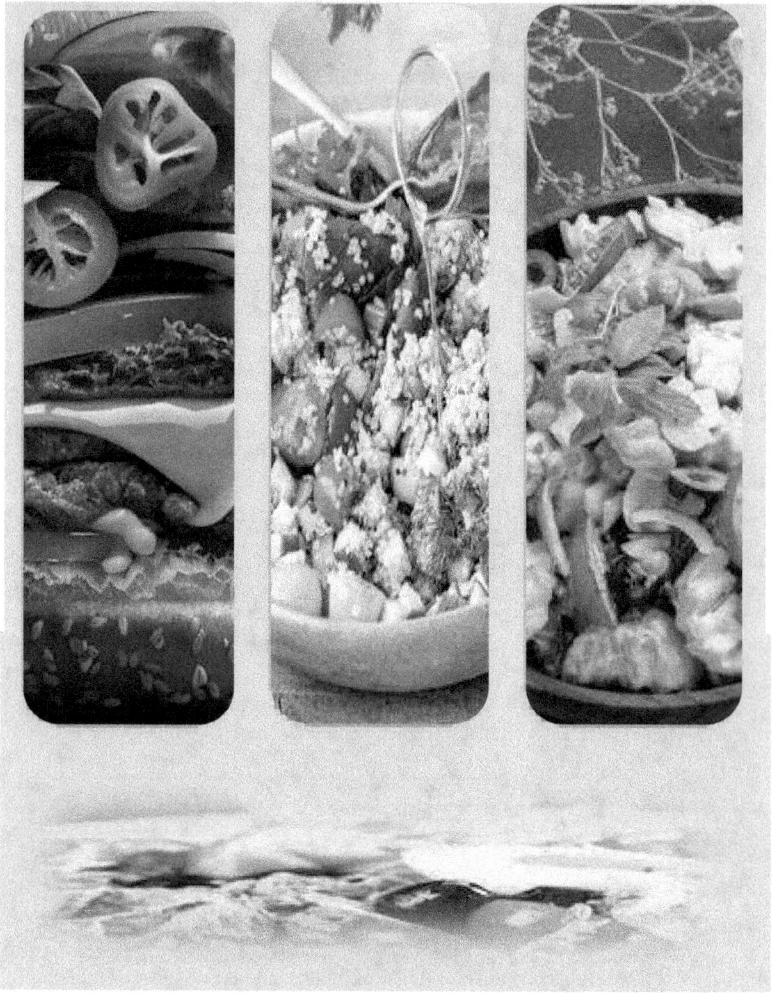

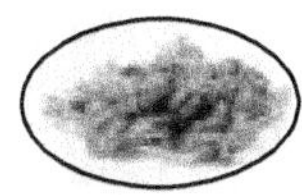 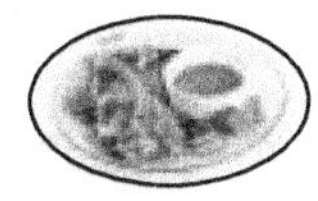 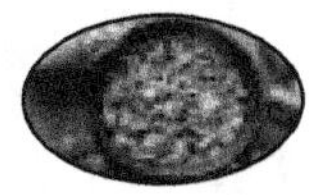

Intrigued, Emily embarked on her own journey into the realm of intermittent fasting. Little did she know that this decision would become a turning point in her life, marking the beginning of a rejuvenated and healthier version of herself.

This book is born from stories like Emily's — tales of resilience, discovery, and transformation. It aims to guide women over a certain age through the intricacies of intermittent fasting, providing a roadmap to reclaim vitality and achieve holistic well-being.

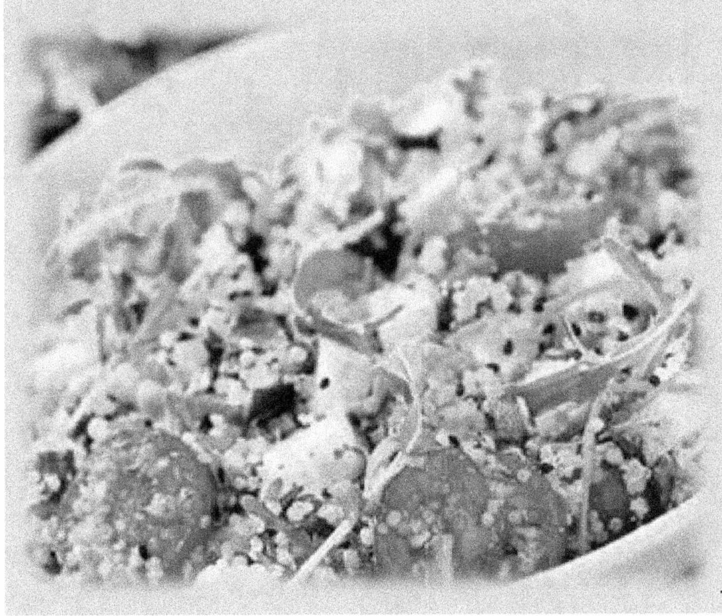

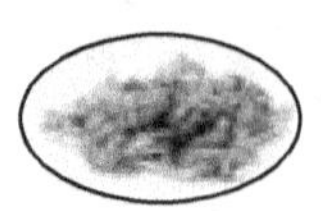 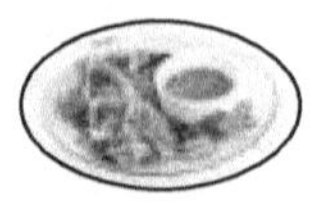 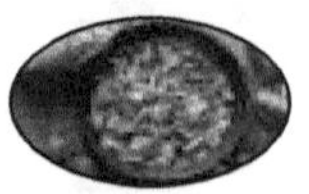

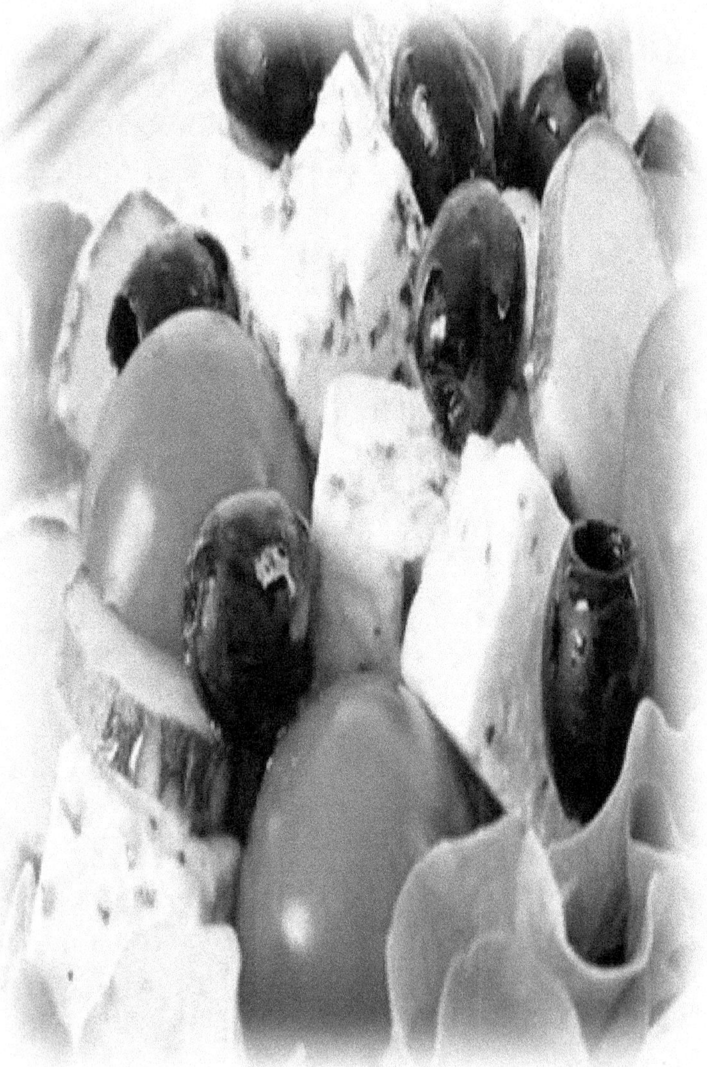

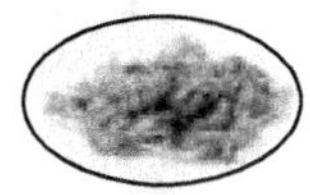 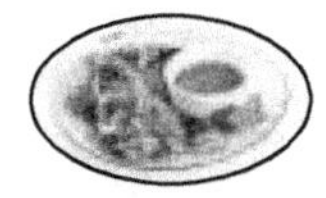 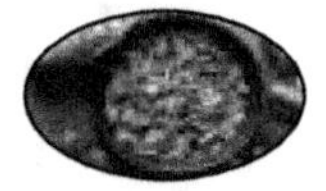

Chapter 1:

Why Intermittent Fasting for Women Over 40

Emily's story is not unique. Many women reaching a certain age find themselves facing unique health challenges — a slowed metabolism, hormonal imbalances, and the stubborn persistence of excess weight. Yet, there is hope in the form of intermittent fasting, a lifestyle change that goes beyond conventional dieting.

1.1 Health Benefits

Intermittent fasting isn't just about shedding pounds; it's a holistic approach to wellness. This chapter delves into the myriad health benefits that make intermittent fasting a compelling choice for women over [specified age].–

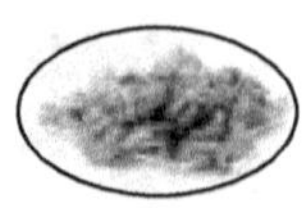 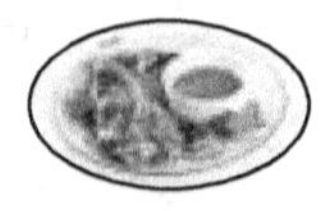 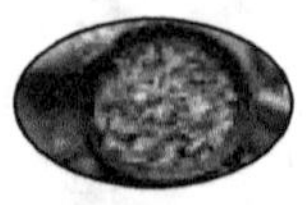

Emily, like many others, discovered that weight management is just the tip of the iceberg. The metabolic reset brought about by intermittent fasting can positively impact hormonal balance, leading to improved mood, reduced inflammation, and enhanced cognitive function.

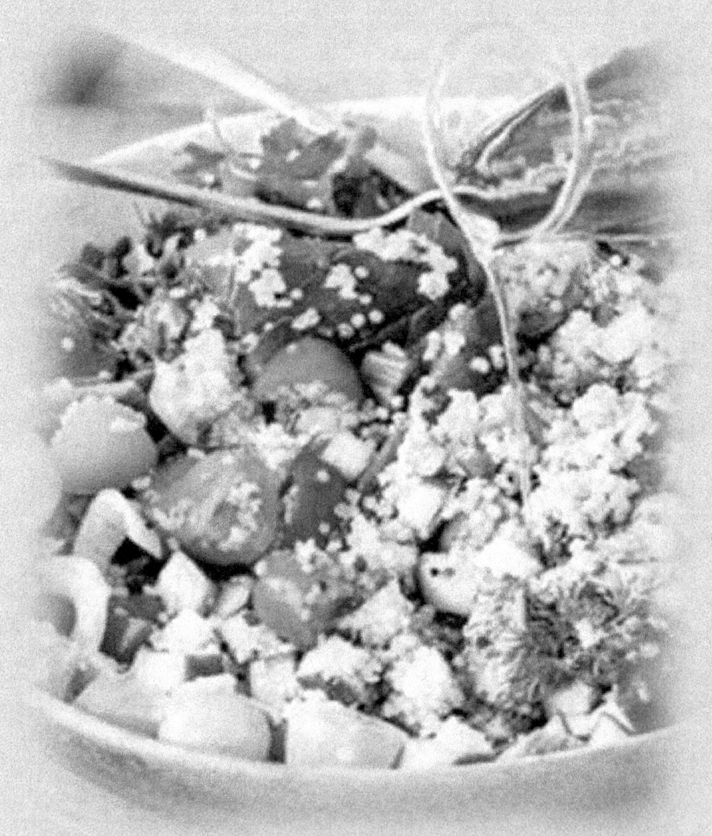

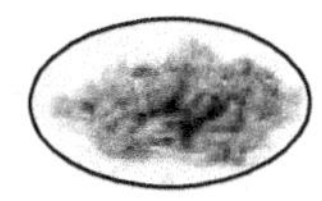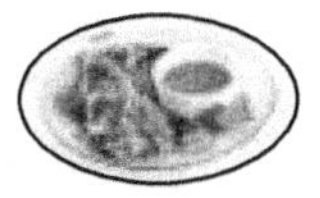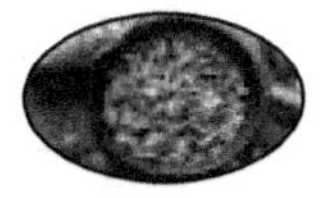

1.2 Tailoring Intermittent Fasting to Women's Needs

Not all fasting approaches are created equal, and women over a certain age require a nuanced strategy. This section explores the importance of tailoring intermittent fasting methods to meet the specific needs and challenges faced by women in this age group.

Understanding that a one-size-fits-all approach doesn't apply, we'll explore different methods such as the 16/8 method, 5:2 method, alternate-day fasting, and other variations. Each method has its own merits, and finding the right fit is crucial for long-term success.

1.3 Setting Realistic Goals

As Emily embarked on her journey, one crucial lesson became apparent: setting realistic goals is the cornerstone of sustainable change. In this section, we'll explore how women over a certain age can establish achievable objectives, fostering a sense of accomplishment and motivation throughout their intermittent fasting adventure.

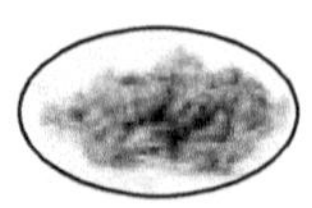 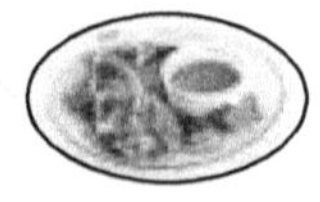 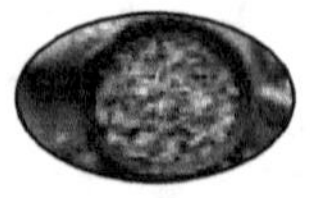

Intermittent fasting is not a sprint; it's a marathon. By understanding the importance of realistic goal-setting, women can create a sustainable plan that aligns with their unique lifestyles and aspirations.

As we unravel the layers of intermittent fasting, it becomes evident that this journey is not just about shedding weight; it's a profound transformation that extends to every facet of a woman's life. In the subsequent chapters, we'll explore the nuts and bolts of getting started, navigating nutrition, overcoming challenges, and ultimately crafting a lifestyle that embraces intermittent fasting for the long haul. Join us on this transformative odyssey towards health, vitality, and a renewed sense of self.

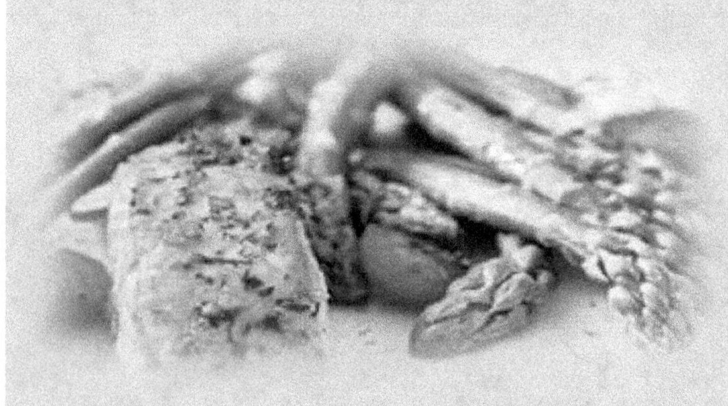

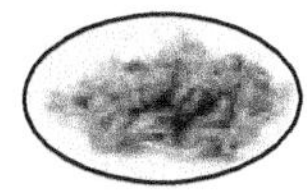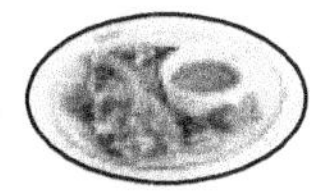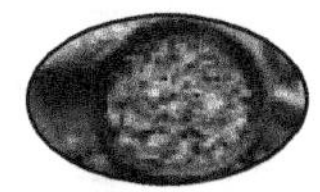

Chapter 2:

In the quaint town of Harmonyville, as Emily delved deeper into the world of intermittent fasting, she realized that the journey ahead was not only about changing eating patterns but embracing a lifestyle that harmonized with her body's needs. Chapter 2 explores the crucial steps for women over a certain age to embark on their own intermittent fasting adventure.

2.1 Consultation with a Healthcare Professional

Before setting sail on the seas of intermittent fasting, it's essential to consult with a healthcare professional. This ensures that individual health needs, potential risks, and any underlying–

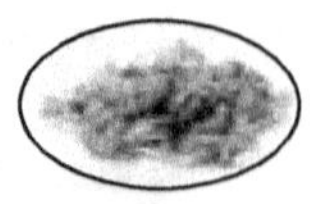 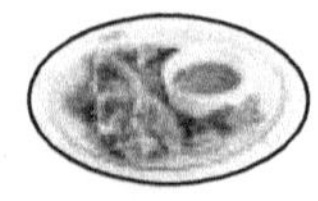 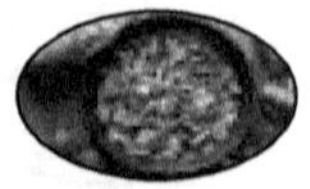

conditions are taken into account. Emily, understanding the importance of this step, scheduled an appointment with her trusted healthcare provider.

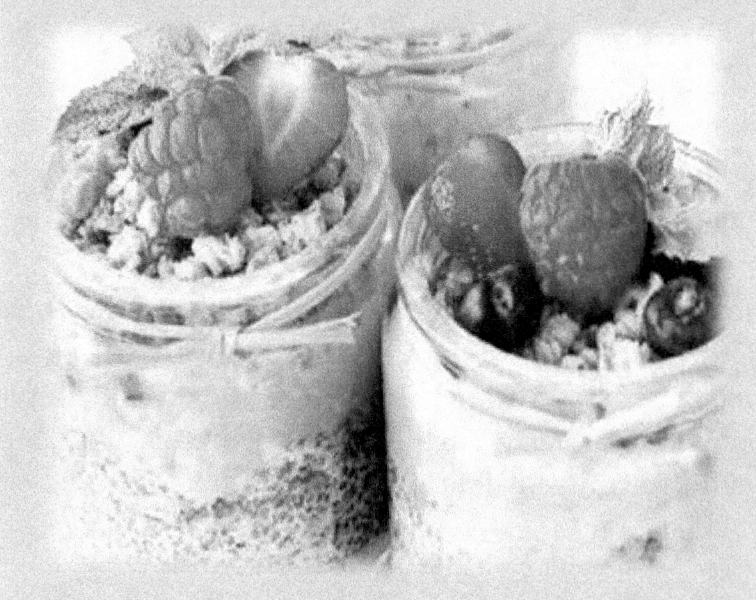

In this section, we emphasize the significance of open communication with healthcare professionals. They can provide personalized advice, monitor progress, and address any concerns that may arise. This collaboration between individuals and their healthcare team forms the bedrock of a safe and effective intermittent fasting journey.–

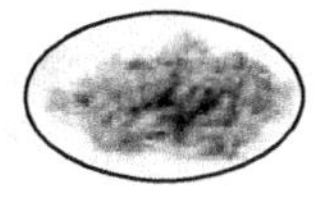 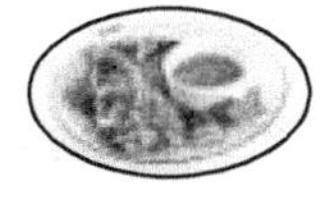 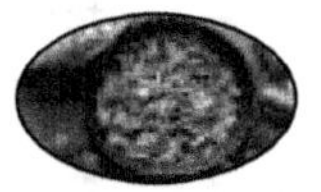

2.2 Choosing the Right Intermittent Fasting Method

With the blessing of her healthcare provider, Emily set out to explore the various intermittent fasting methods. This section provides an in-depth look at popular methods, helping women over a certain age choose the one that aligns with their preferences and lifestyle.

- *16/8 Method*: A daily fasting window of 16 hours with an 8-hour eating window.

- *5:2 Method*: Alternating between normal eating and two days of reduced calorie intake.

- *Alternate-Day Fasting*: Cycling between days of regular eating and days of fasting.

By understanding the intricacies of each method, women can make informed decisions that suit their unique circumstances. Flexibility is key, and the goal is to find a method that promotes adherence and long-term success.–

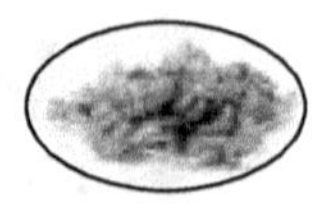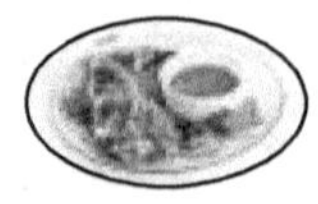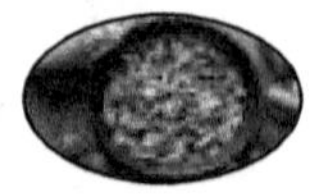

2.3 Setting Realistic Goals

As Emily discussed her chosen fasting method with her healthcare provider, they collaboratively set realistic goals tailored to her age, health status, and lifestyle. This section emphasizes the importance of establishing clear, achievable objectives.

Whether the goal is weight loss, improved energy levels, or enhanced mental clarity, having a roadmap in place ensures that the intermittent fasting journey remains focused and purposeful. Realistic goals act as beacons of progress, motivating women to stay committed to their chosen path.

2.4 Embracing Mindfulness

Intermittent fasting isn't solely about what you eat but also about how you approach food. Mindful eating plays a crucial role in this journey, fostering a deeper connection with the body's hunger and satiety cues.–

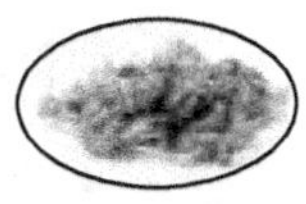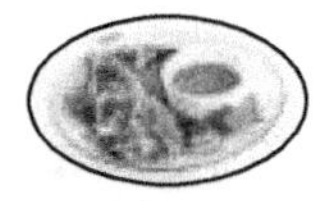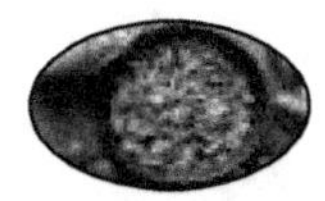

In this section, we explore the concept of mindful eating — savoring each bite, recognizing true hunger, and being attuned to the body's signals. Emily found that embracing mindfulness transformed her relationship with food, making her intermittent fasting experience more enriching and sustainable.

2.5 Navigating Social Situations

One of the challenges Emily faced was navigating social situations while adhering to her chosen intermittent fasting method. This section provides practical tips on how women over a certain age can maintain their fasting routine without feeling isolated during social gatherings.

From communicating their dietary choices with friends and family to planning social events around eating windows, these strategies empower women to strike a balance between their social lives and intermittent fasting commitments.

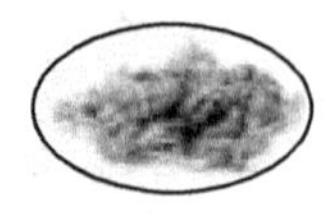 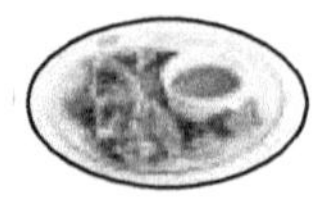 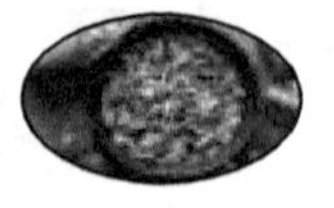

As Emily progressed in her intermittent fasting journey, she learned that adaptability is key. This section discusses how women can adjust their fasting schedules based on life's changing demands, ensuring that intermittent fasting remains a sustainable and dynamic lifestyle choice.

Whether it's adapting to travel, changes in work schedules, or personal commitments, the ability to adjust the fasting schedule promotes long-term adherence and prevents the feeling of being confined by rigid rules.

Embarking on the intermittent fasting journey requires thoughtful planning, collaboration with healthcare professionals, and the cultivation of a mindful and adaptable mindset. In the upcoming chapters, we'll delve into the critical aspects of nutrition, exercise, and hormonal considerations, providing a comprehensive guide for women over a certain age to unlock the full potential of intermittent fasting and transform their lives. Join us as we continue this transformative odyssey towards health and well-being.–

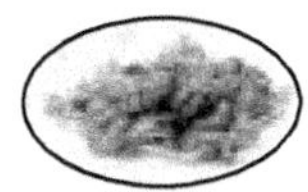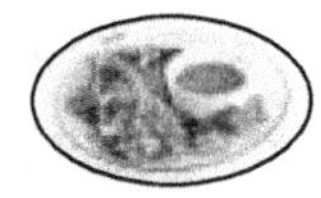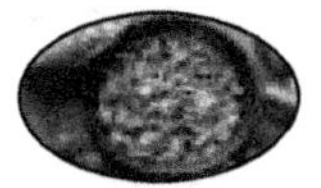

Chapter 3:

In the heart of Harmonyville, as Emily embraced the rhythm of intermittent fasting, she quickly realized that success went beyond the timing of meals. Nutrition became the cornerstone of her journey, shaping not only what she ate but how she nourished her body during eating windows. Chapter 3 explores the intricate dance between intermittent fasting and nutrition for women over a certain age.

3.1 Importance of Nutrient-Rich Foods

As Emily took her first steps into the world of intermittent fasting, she discovered the profound impact of nutrient-rich foods on overall well-being. This section emphasizes the importance of prioritizing nutrient-dense, whole foods to support health and vitality.

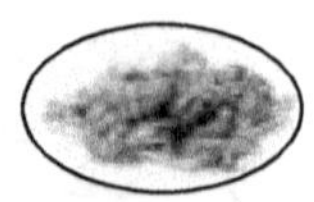 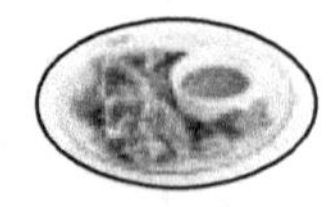 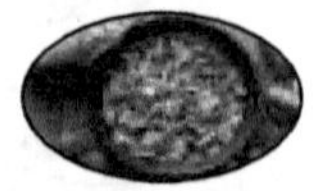

From leafy greens and colorful vegetables to lean proteins and healthy fats, the body benefits from a diverse range of nutrients. Ensuring an ample supply of vitamins, minerals, and antioxidants becomes paramount, as these elements play key roles in energy metabolism, hormonal balance, and immune function.

3.2 Micronutrient Considerations

Women over a certain age often face unique nutritional needs, particularly concerning micronutrients like calcium, vitamin D, and iron. In this section, we delve into the specific micronutrient considerations that should be addressed during intermittent fasting to support bone health, immune function, and overall vitality.

Emily, recognizing the significance of micronutrients, incorporated a variety of foods into her meals to ensure a well-rounded nutritional profile. The exploration of micronutrient-rich options becomes a crucial aspect of meal planning for women embracing intermittent fasting.–

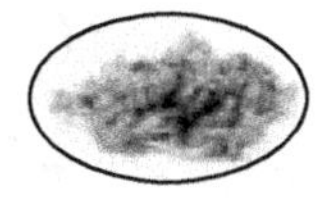 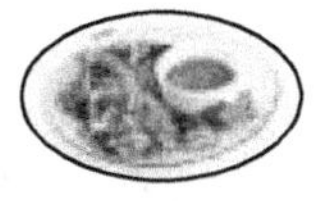 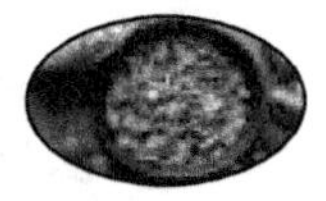

3.3 Balancing Macronutrients

The balance of macronutrients — carbohydrates, proteins, and fats — plays a pivotal role in the effectiveness of intermittent fasting. Women over a certain age need to strike a balance that aligns with their health goals, supporting energy levels and hormonal balance.

This section guides readers through the principles of macronutrient balance, helping them understand the role of each component in the body's functioning. Tailoring the macronutrient distribution to individual needs ensures that women derive maximum benefit from their intermittent fasting journey.

3.4 Sample Meal Plans

Practicality is key in sustaining any lifestyle change, and intermittent fasting is no exception. This section provides sample meal plans tailored to different intermittent fasting methods, offering a glimpse into what a day of balanced eating might look like.–

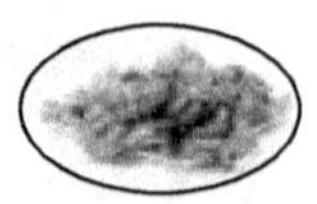 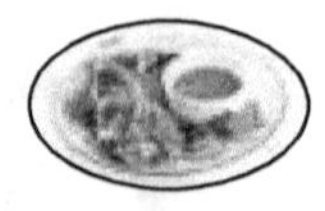 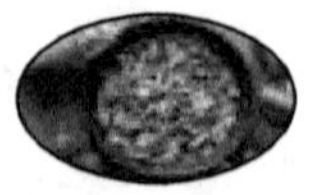

From breakfast ideas for those following the 16/8 method to strategies for managing calorie intake on fasting days in the 5:2 method, these sample meal plans serve as valuable guides. Emily, drawing inspiration from such plans, found the flexibility to craft meals that suited her tastes while adhering to her chosen fasting routine.

3.5 Hydration during Fasting Periods

As Emily embraced intermittent fasting, she discovered that staying well-hydrated was as crucial as mindful eating. This section explores the importance of hydration during fasting periods and provides practical tips for ensuring adequate water intake.

Whether through herbal teas, infused water, or simply sipping on plain water, maintaining hydration supports metabolic function and helps mitigate feelings of hunger. Emily, armed with a water bottle by her side, found that staying hydrated enhanced her overall well-being during intermittent fasting.–

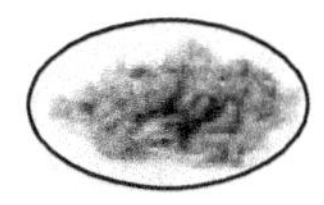 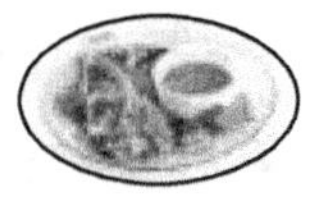 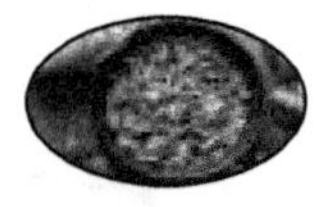

3.6 Intermittent Fasting and Gut Health

A healthy gut is the foundation of overall well-being, and intermittent fasting can influence gut health positively. This section delves into the relationship between intermittent fasting and gut health, exploring how fasting periods may contribute to a balanced and thriving gut microbiome.

From incorporating probiotic-rich foods to being mindful of prebiotics, women over a certain age can nurture their gut health alongside their intermittent fasting journey. Emily, experiencing improved digestion and gut comfort, realized the interconnectedness of her dietary choices and overall wellness.

3.7 Mindful Eating Practices

In the hustle and bustle of everyday life, mindful eating often takes a backseat. This section encourages women to slow down, savor each bite, and cultivate mindful eating practices. Emily discovered that being present during meals not

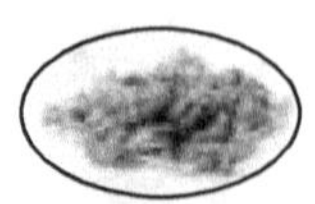 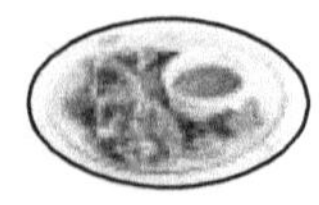 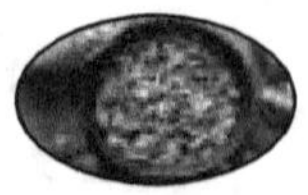

only enhanced her enjoyment of food but also helped her tune in to her body's hunger and fullness cues.

Mindful eating is a powerful tool that aligns seamlessly with intermittent fasting, fostering a deeper connection between individuals and their dietary choices. By embracing mindful eating practices, women can enrich their intermittent fasting experience and foster a healthier relationship with food.

Navigating the intricacies of nutrition during intermittent fasting is a vital aspect of the journey. As we continue to unravel the layers of this transformative lifestyle, the upcoming chapters will explore strategies for overcoming challenges, incorporating exercise, and addressing hormonal considerations. Join us as we navigate the path to wellness, armed with knowledge and empowered to make informed choices in the realm of nutrition and meal planning.–

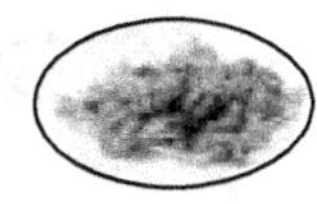 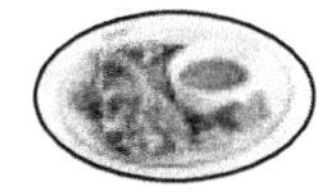 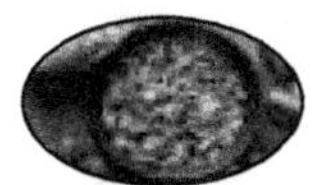

Green Smoothie Delight

Ingredients:

- 1 cup spinach leaves

- 1/2 cucumber, peeled and sliced

- 1/2 avocado, peeled and pitted

- 1/2 green apple, cored and chopped

- 1 tablespoon chia seeds

- 1 cup water or almond milk

Instructions:

1. Combine all ingredients in a blender.

2. Blend until smooth.

3. Pour into a glass and enjoy!–

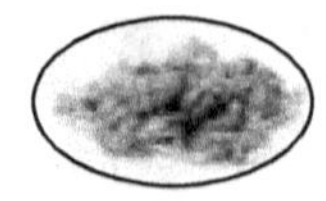 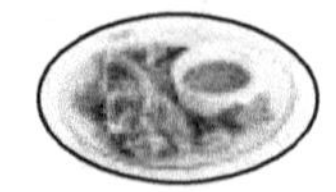 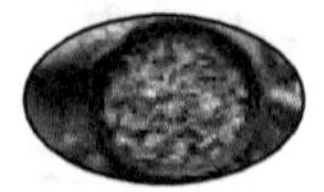

Protein-Packed Egg Muffins

Ingredients:

- 4 eggs

- 1/2 cup diced bell peppers

- 1/2 cup diced tomatoes

- 1/4 cup diced onions

- 1/2 cup spinach, chopped

- Salt and pepper to taste

Instructions:

1. Preheat oven to 350°F (175°C).

2. In a bowl, beat eggs and add vegetables.

3. Season with salt and pepper.

4. Pour mixture into muffin tin.

5. Bake for 20 minutes or until eggs are set.–

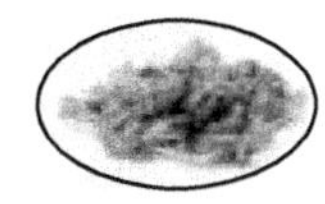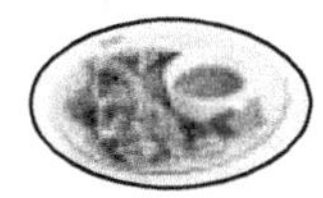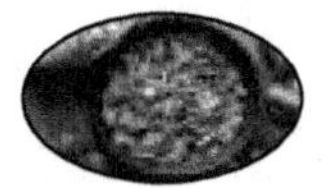

Berry Bliss Yogurt Parfait

Ingredients:

- 1 cup Greek yogurt

- 1/2 cup of berry mixture (raspberries, blueberries, and strawberries)

- 1 tablespoon honey

- 2 tablespoons granola

Instructions:

1. In a glass, layer yogurt, berries, and granola.

2. Drizzle honey on top.

3. Repeat layers.

4. Enjoy this delicious parfait!–

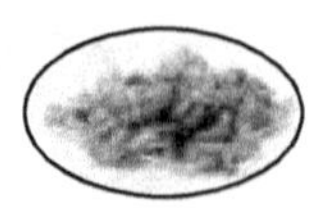 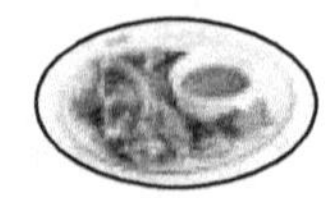 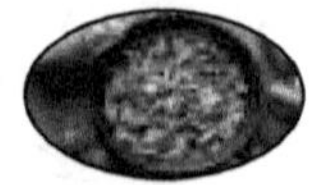

Grilled Chicken Salad

Ingredients:

- 4 oz grilled chicken breast, sliced

- 2 cups mixed salad greens

- 1/2 cup cherry tomatoes, halved

- 1/4 cup sliced cucumber

- 1 tablespoon olive oil

- 1 tablespoon balsamic vinegar

Instructions:

1. Combine chicken, salad greens, tomatoes, and cucumber in a bowl.

2. Whisk together olive oil and balsamic vinegar for dressing.

3. Toss salad with dressing and serve.–

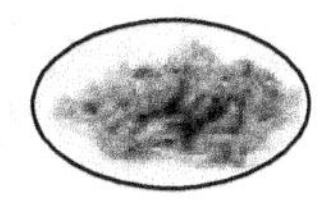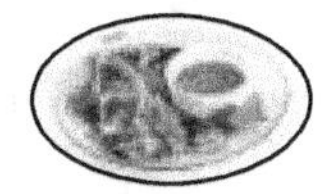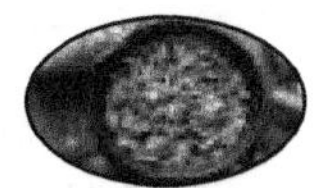

Quinoa Veggie Bowl

Ingredients:

- 1 cup cooked quinoa

- Half a cup of rinsed and drained black beans

- 1/2 cup corn kernels

- 1/2 cup diced bell peppers

- 1/4 cup chopped cilantro

- 1 tablespoon lime juice

Instructions:

1. In a bowl, mix quinoa, black beans, corn, bell peppers, cilantro, and lime juice.

2. Stir well and enjoy this nutritious bowl.–

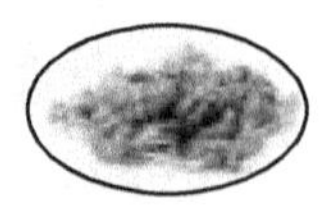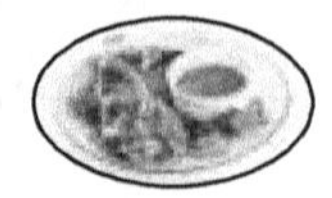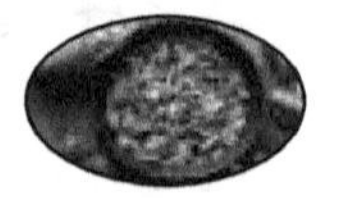

Salmon and Asparagus Foil Pack

Ingredients:

- 4 oz salmon fillet

- 1 cup asparagus, trimmed

- 1 tablespoon olive oil

- Lemon slices

- Salt and pepper to taste

Instructions:

1. Preheat oven to 375°F (190°C).

2. Place salmon and asparagus on a piece of foil.

3. Drizzle with olive oil, add lemon slices, and season with salt and pepper.

4. Seal the foil and bake for 20 minutes.–

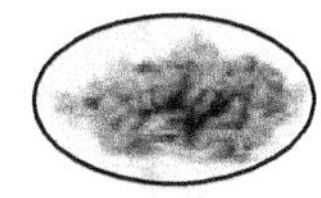 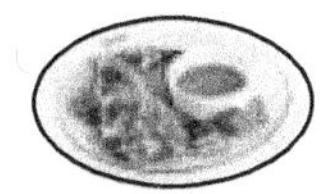 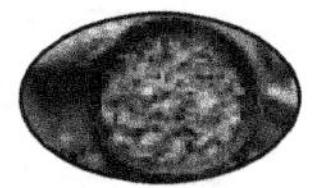

Avocado and Turkey Wrap

Ingredients:

- 1 whole wheat tortilla

- 2 oz turkey slices

- 1/2 avocado, sliced

- Handful of spinach leaves

- 1 tablespoon Greek yogurt

Instructions:

1. Lay tortilla flat and layer with turkey, avocado, spinach, and Greek yogurt.

2. Roll tightly and slice in half for a satisfying wrap.

Sweet Potato and Chickpea Hash

Ingredients:

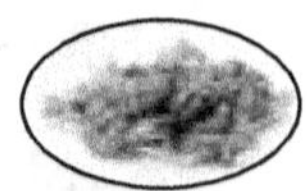 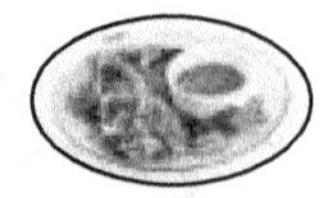 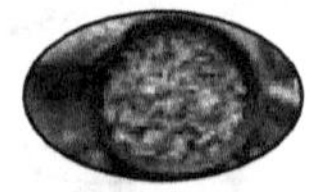

- 1 medium sweet potato, diced

- 1/2 can chickpeas, drained and rinsed

- 1/2 red onion, chopped

- 1 teaspoon olive oil

- 1/2 teaspoon cumin

- Salt and pepper to taste

Instructions:

1. Heat olive oil in a pan and sauté sweet potato, chickpeas, and red onion.

2. Season with cumin, salt, and pepper.

3. Cook until sweet potatoes are tender.

Recipe 9:

Cucumber and Tuna Bites

Ingredients:

- 1 cucumber, sliced

- 1 can tuna, drained

- 1 tablespoon mayonnaise

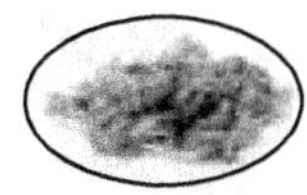 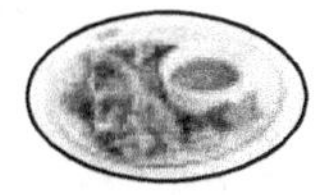 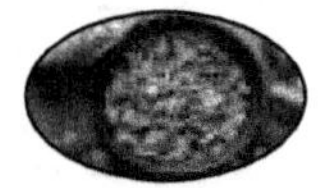

- 1 teaspoon Dijon mustard

- Salt and pepper to taste

Instructions:

1. Mix tuna, mayonnaise, and Dijon mustard in a bowl.

2. Spoon onto cucumber slices.

3. Sprinkle with salt and pepper.

Recipe 10:

Berry Almond Chia Pudding

Ingredients:

- 1/4 cup chia seeds

- 1 cup almond milk

- 1/2 cup mixed berries

- 1 tablespoon almond slices

- 1 teaspoon honey–

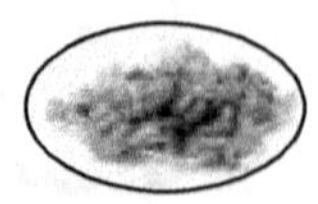 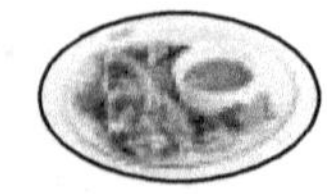 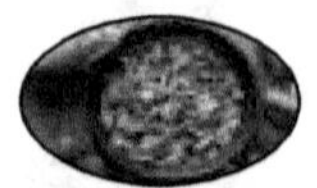

Instructions:

1. Mix chia seeds and almond milk in a jar, refrigerate overnight.

2. In the morning, layer chia pudding with berries and almond slices.

3. Drizzle honey on top and savor this delightful pudding.

Recipe 11:

Veggie Omelette

Ingredients:

- 3 eggs

- 1/4 cup diced bell peppers

- 1/4 cup diced tomatoes

- 1/4 cup chopped spinach

- 1/4 cup shredded cheese

- Salt and pepper to taste–

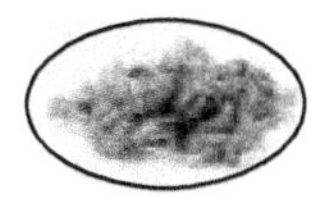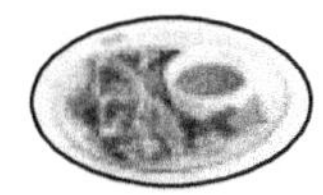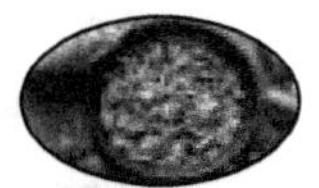

Instructions:

1. Whisk eggs and pour into a heated, oiled pan.

2. Add bell peppers, tomatoes, spinach, and cheese on one half.

3. Fold the omelette in half and cook until the cheese melts.

Zucchini Noodles with Pesto

Ingredients:

- 2 medium zucchinis, spiralized
- 1/4 cup cherry tomatoes, halved
- 2 tablespoons pesto sauce
- 1 tablespoon grated Parmesan cheese

Instructions:

1. Sauté zucchini noodles in a pan until tender.

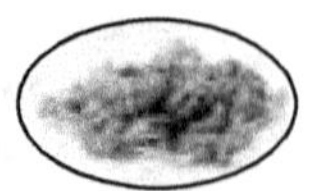 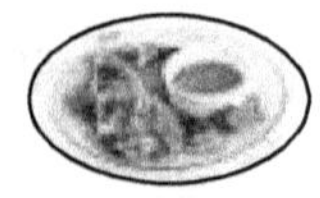 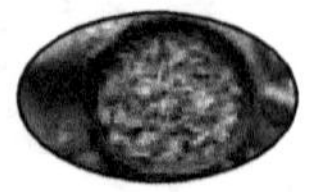

2. Toss with cherry tomatoes, pesto, and Parmesan cheese.

3. Serve for a light and flavorful meal.

Greek Salad Skewers

Ingredients:

- Cherry tomatoes

- Cucumber, cut into chunks

- Feta cheese, cubed

- Kalamata olives

- Olive oil and oregano for drizzling

Instructions:

1. Thread tomatoes, cucumber, feta, and olives onto skewers.

2. Sprinkle oregano over top and drizzle with olive oil.–

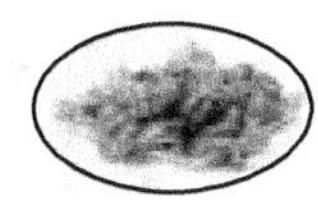 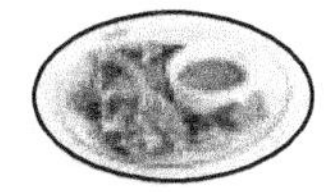 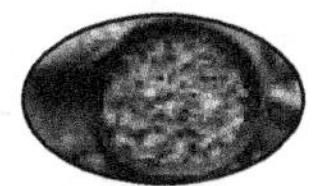

Turkey and Veggie Stir-Fry

Ingredients:

- 1/2 lb ground turkey

- 1 cup broccoli florets

- 1/2 cup sliced bell peppers

- 1/4 cup soy sauce

- 1 tablespoon sesame oil

Instructions:

1. Brown turkey in a pan, add vegetables, and stir-fry.

2. Mix in soy sauce and sesame oil.

3. Serve over cauliflower rice for a low-carb option.–

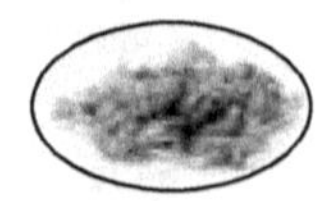 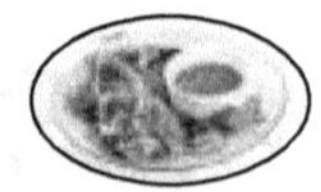 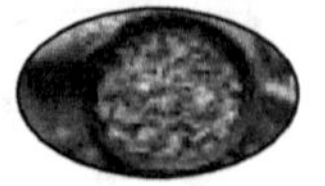

Cauliflower Pizza Crust

Ingredients:

- 1 medium cauliflower, grated
- 1 egg
- 1/2 cup grated mozzarella cheese
- 1 teaspoon Italian seasoning
- Tomato sauce and desired toppings

Instructions:

1. Mix cauliflower, egg, cheese, and seasoning.

2. Press into a crust shape and bake at 400°F (200°C) for 20 minutes.

3. Add sauce and toppings, bake until cheese melts.–

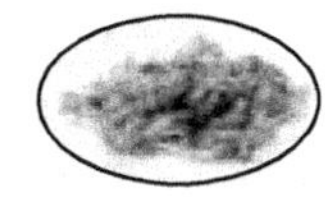 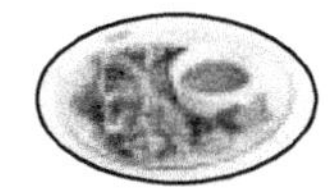 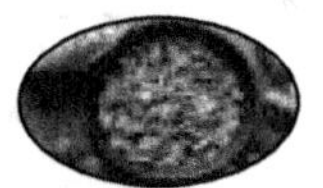

Almond Butter Banana Bites

Ingredients:

- Banana slices

- Almond butter

- Chia seeds

- Honey for drizzling

Instructions:

1. Spread almond butter on banana slices.

2. Sprinkle with chia seeds.

3. Drizzle with honey for a sweet and satisfying treat.

Caprese Salad

Ingredients:

- Fresh mozzarella, sliced

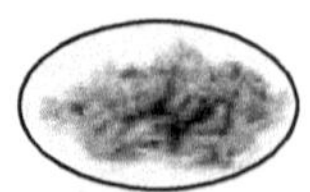 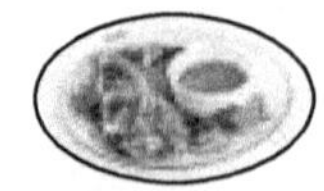 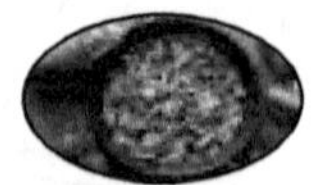

- Tomatoes, sliced

- Fresh basil leaves

- Balsamic glaze

- Salt and pepper to taste

Instructions:

1. Arrange mozzarella, tomatoes, and basil on a plate.

2. Drizzle with balsamic glaze, season with salt and pepper.

Recipe 18:

Lentil Soup

Ingredients:

- 1 cup dried lentils

- 1/2 onion, diced

- 2 carrots, sliced

- 2 celery stalks, chopped

- 4 cups vegetable broth

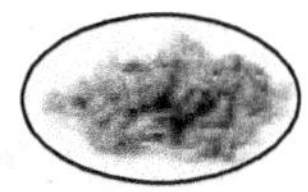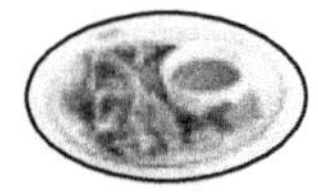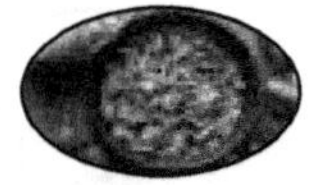

- 1 teaspoon cumin

- Salt and pepper to taste

Instructions:

1. Rinse lentils and combine with vegetables, broth, and spices in a pot.

2. Simmer until lentils are tender.

Turkey Lettuce Wraps

Ingredients:

- 1/2 lb ground turkey

- 1/2 cup diced water chestnuts

- 1/4 cup hoisin sauce

- Lettuce leaves for wrapping

Instructions:

1. Brown turkey, add water chestnuts, and stir in hoisin sauce.

2. Spoon into lettuce leaves for a light and flavorful wrap.

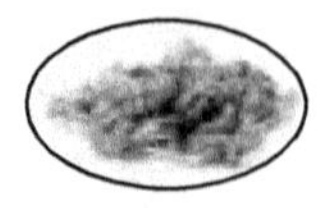 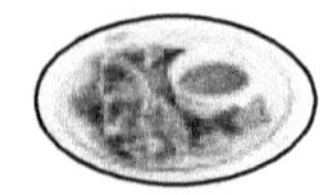 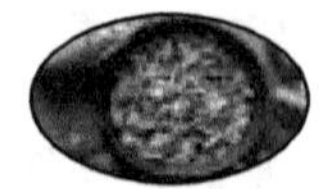

Mango Coconut Chia Popsicles

Ingredients:

- 1 cup mango chunks

- 1 cup coconut milk

- 2 tablespoons chia seeds

- 1 tablespoon honey

Instructions:

1. Blend mango and coconut milk until smooth.

2. Stir in chia seeds and honey.

3. Pour into popsicle molds and freeze. Enjoy your refreshing popsicles!–

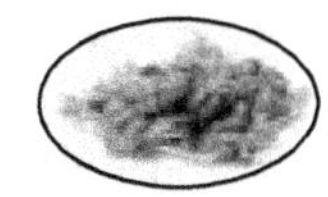 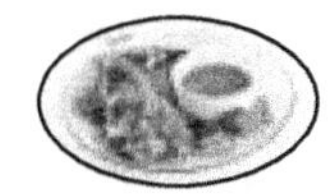 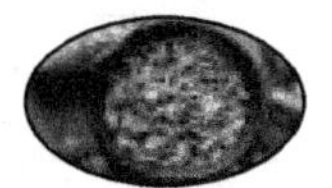

Shrimp and Broccoli Stir-Fry

Ingredients:

- 1/2 lb shrimp, peeled and deveined
- 2 cups broccoli florets
- 1/4 cup soy sauce
- 1 tablespoon ginger, minced
- 2 cloves garlic, minced

Instructions:

1. Sauté shrimp in a pan until pink.
2. Add broccoli, soy sauce, ginger, and garlic.
3. Stir-fry broccoli until it becomes soft.

Spinach and Feta Stuffed Chicken Breast

Ingredients:

- 2 boneless, skinless chicken breasts

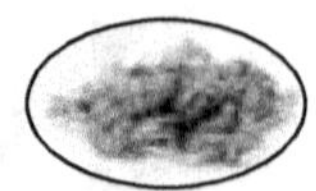 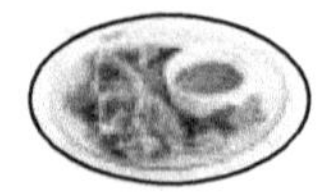 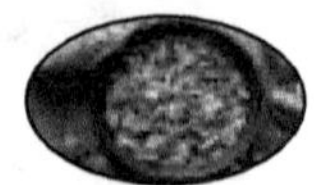

- 1 cup fresh spinach

- 1/4 cup feta cheese, crumbled

- 1 teaspoon Italian seasoning

- Salt and pepper to taste

Instructions:

1. Preheat oven to 400°F (200°C).

2. Butterfly chicken breasts and stuff with spinach and feta.

3. Season with Italian seasoning, salt, and pepper.

4. Bake for 25-30 minutes or until chicken is cooked through.

Recipe 23:

Avocado Tuna Salad

Ingredients:

- 1 can tuna, drained

- 1 avocado, mashed

- 1/4 red onion, finely diced

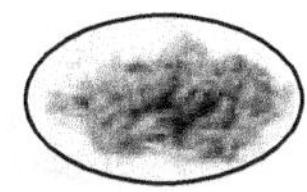 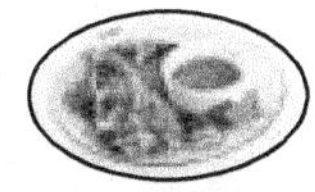 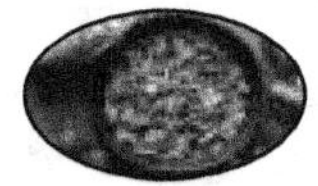

- 1 tablespoon mayonnaise

- Salt and pepper to taste

Instructions:

1. Mix tuna, mashed avocado, red onion, and mayonnaise.

2. Season with salt and pepper.

3. Serve on lettuce leaves or whole grain crackers.

Broccoli and Cheese Stuffed Portobello Mushrooms

Ingredients:

- 4 large portobello mushrooms

- 2 cups broccoli florets, steamed

- 1 cup shredded cheddar cheese

- 2 tablespoons olive oil

- Salt and pepper to taste–

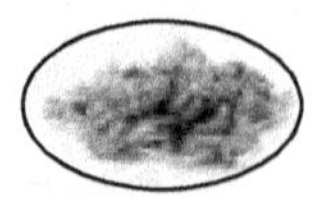 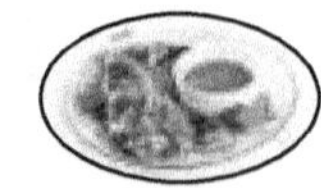 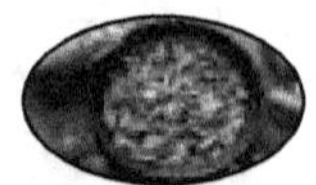

Instructions:

1. Remove stems from mushrooms and brush with olive oil.

2. Fill mushrooms with steamed broccoli and top with cheese.

3. Bake at 375°F (190°C) for 15-20 minutes.

Cauliflower Fried Rice

Ingredients:

- 1 head cauliflower, grated

- 1/2 cup diced carrots

- 1/2 cup peas

- 2 eggs, beaten

- 2 tablespoons soy sauce

Instructions:

1. Sauté cauliflower, carrots, and peas in a pan.

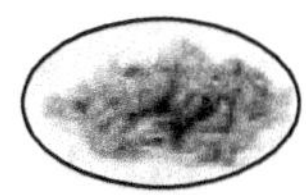 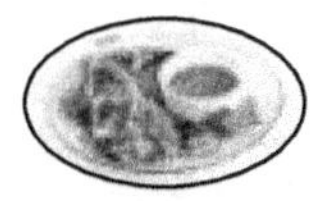 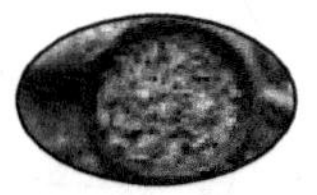

2. Push vegetables to the side, pour beaten eggs, and scramble.

3. Mix everything together, add soy sauce, and stir-fry.

Turkey and Vegetable Skewers

Ingredients:

- 1/2 lb turkey breast, cubed

- Cherry tomatoes

- Bell peppers, cut into chunks

- Red onion, sliced

- Olive oil and herbs for marinade

Instructions:

1. Marinate turkey in olive oil and herbs.

2. Thread turkey, tomatoes, peppers, and onion onto skewers.

3. Grill until turkey is cooked through.–

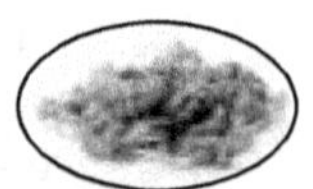 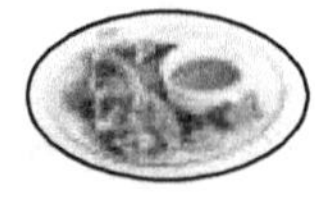 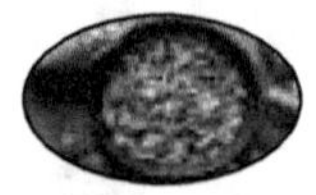

Recipe 27: Chocolate Avocado Mousse

Ingredients:

- 2 ripe avocados
- 1/4 cup cocoa powder
- 1/4 cup maple syrup
- 1 teaspoon vanilla extract

Instructions:

1. Until smooth, blend avocados, cocoa powder, maple syrup, and vanilla.

2. Allow it cool in the fridge for a minimum of one hour.

3. Serve as a dessert without guilt.

Recipe 28:

Mediterranean Chickpea Salad

Ingredients:

- 1 can chickpeas, drained
- Cucumber, diced

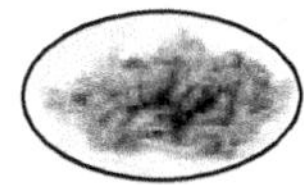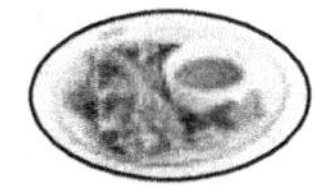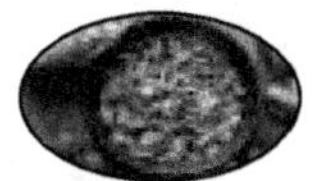

- Cherry tomatoes, halved

- Red onion, finely chopped

- Feta cheese, crumbled

- Olive oil and lemon juice dressing

Instructions:

1. Combine chickpeas, cucumber, tomatoes, onion, and feta in a bowl.

2. Pour in some lemon juice and olive oil.

3. Toss and enjoy this refreshing salad.

Recipe 29:

Eggplant Parmesan

Ingredients:

- 1 large eggplant, sliced

- 1 cup marinara sauce

- 1 cup mozzarella cheese, shredded

- 1/2 cup grated Parmesan cheese

- Fresh basil for garnish

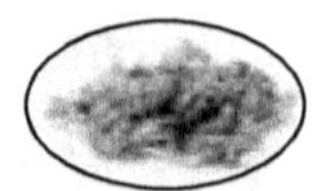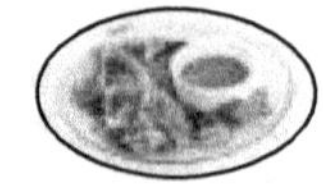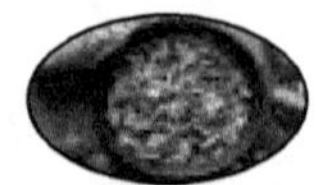

Instructions:

1. Bake eggplant slices until golden.

2. Layer in a baking dish with marinara sauce and cheeses.

3. Bake until cheese is bubbly. Garnish with fresh basil.

Blueberry Almond Chia Smoothie

Ingredients:

- 1/2 cup blueberries

- 1 cup almond milk

- 1 tablespoon almond butter

- 1 tablespoon chia seeds

- Ice cubes

Instructions:

1. Blend blueberries, almond milk, almond butter, and chia seeds until smooth.

2. Add ice cubes and blend again.

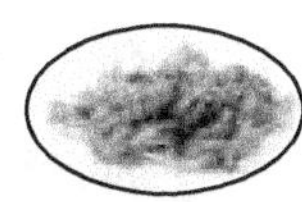 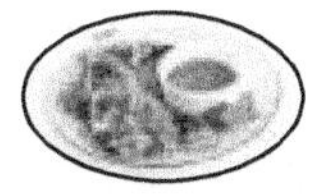 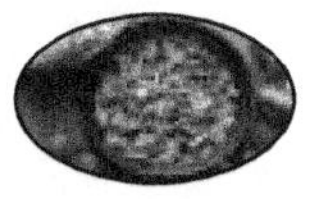

3. Pour into a glass and enjoy this nutritious smoothie.

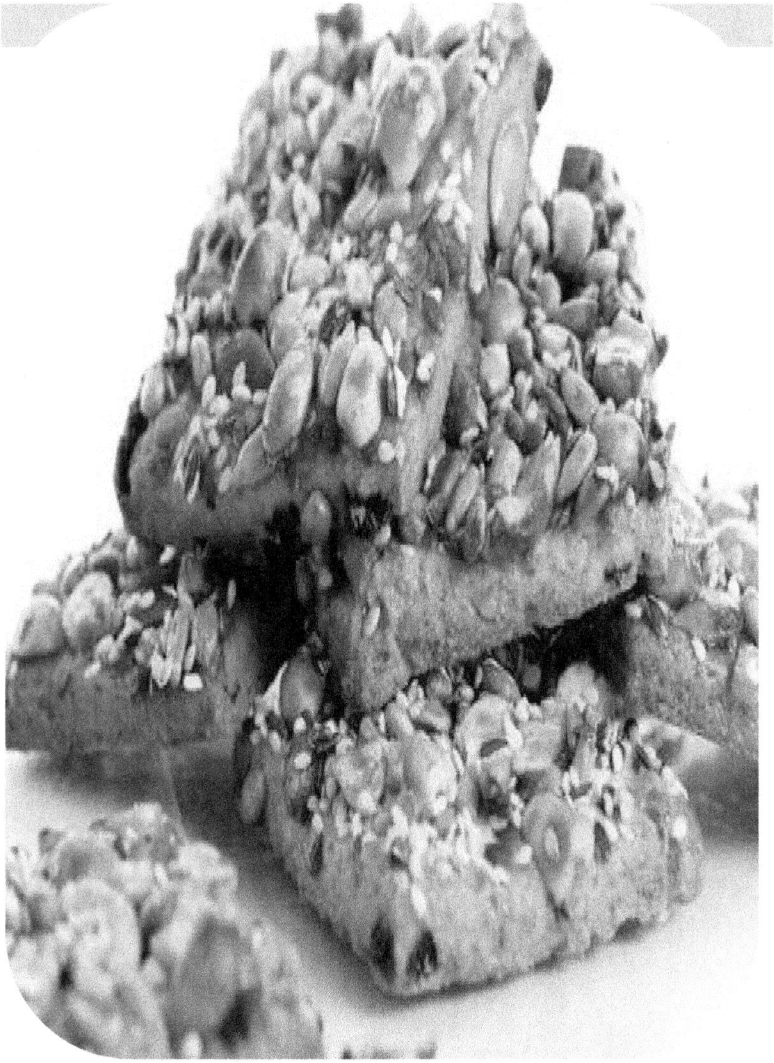

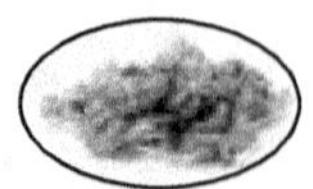 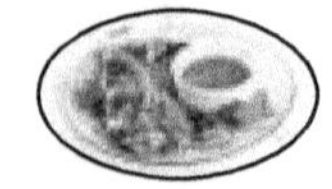 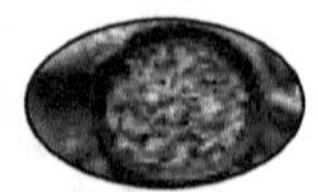

28-Day Intermittent Fasting Meal Plan

Day 1:

- **Breakfast:** Green Smoothie Delight
- **Lunch:** Quinoa Veggie Bowl
- **Dinner:** Grilled Chicken Salad

Day 2:

- **Breakfast:** Protein-Packed Egg Muffins
- **Lunch:** Turkey and Vegetable Skewers
- **Dinner:** Broccoli and Cheese Stuffed Portobello Mushrooms–

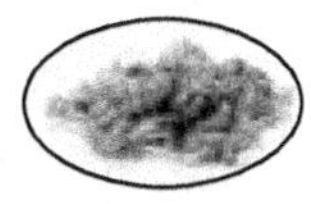 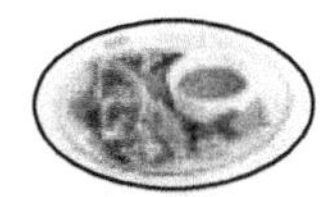 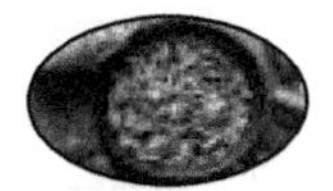

Day 3:

- **Breakfast:** Berry Bliss Yogurt Parfait

- **Lunch:** Cauliflower Fried Rice

- **Dinner:** Mediterranean Chickpea Salad

Day 4:

- **Breakfast:** Avocado Tuna Salad

- **Lunch:** Blueberry Almond Chia Smoothie

- **Dinner:** Shrimp and Broccoli Stir-Fry

Day 5:

- **Breakfast:** Chocolate Avocado Mousse

- **Lunch:** Turkey Lettuce Wraps

- **Dinner:** Eggplant Parmesan–

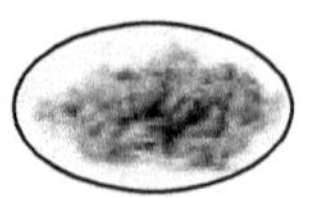 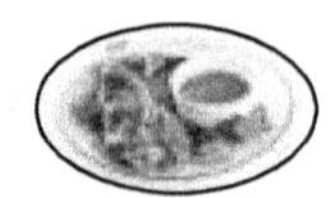 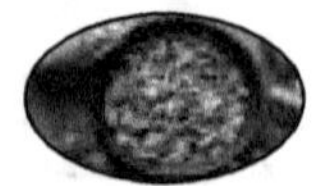

Day 6:

- **Breakfast:** Mango Coconut Chia Popsicles

- **Lunch:** Caprese Salad

- **Dinner:** Sweet Potato and Chickpea Hash

Day 7:

- **Breakfast:** Zucchini Noodles with Pesto

- **Lunch:** Lentil Soup

- **Dinner:** Salmon and Asparagus Foil Pack

Day 8:

- **Breakfast:** Spinach and Feta Stuffed Chicken Breast

- **Lunch:** Cucumber and Tuna Bites

- **Dinner:** Veggie Omelette

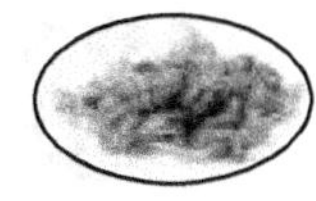 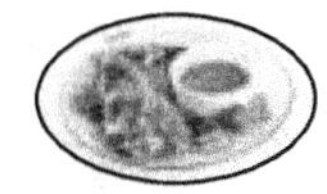 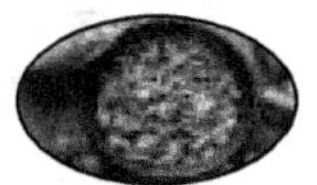

- **Breakfast:** Almond Butter Banana Bites
- **Lunch:** Greek Salad Skewers
- **Dinner:** Berry Almond Chia Pudding

- **Breakfast:** Avocado and Turkey Wrap
- **Lunch:** Shrimp and Broccoli Stir-Fry
- **Dinner:** Quinoa Veggie Bowl

- **Breakfast:** Protein-Packed Egg Muffins
- **Lunch:** Broccoli and Cheese Stuffed Portobello Mushrooms
- **Dinner:** Grilled Chicken Salad

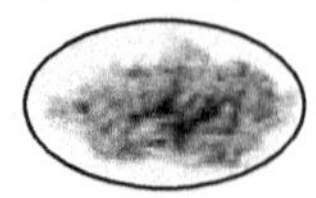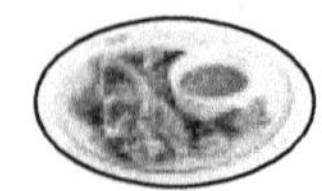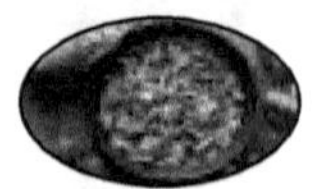

Day 12:

- **Breakfast:** Berry Bliss Yogurt Parfait

- **Lunch:** Caprese Salad

- **Dinner:** Sweet Potato and Chickpea Hash

Day 13:

- **Breakfast:** Chocolate Avocado Mousse

- **Lunch:** Mediterranean Chickpea Salad

- **Dinner:** Salmon and Asparagus Foil Pack

Day 14:

- **Breakfast:** Mango Coconut Chia Popsicles

- **Lunch:** Turkey Lettuce Wraps

- **Dinner:** Eggplant Parmesan

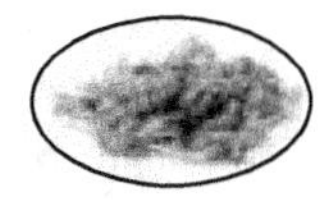 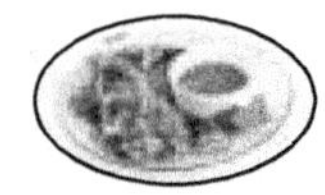 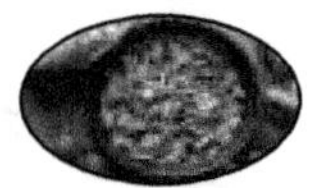

Day 15:

- **Breakfast:** Zucchini Noodles with Pesto

- **Lunch:** Cucumber and Tuna Bites

- **Dinner:** Veggie Omelette

Day 16:

- **Breakfast:** Almond Butter Banana Bites

- **Lunch:** Lentil Soup

- **Dinner:** Berry Almond Chia Pudding

Day 17:

- **Breakfast:** Avocado and Turkey Wrap

- **Lunch:** Shrimp and Broccoli Stir-Fry

- **Dinner:** Quinoa Veggie Bowl

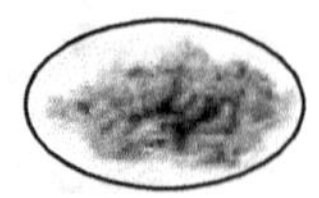 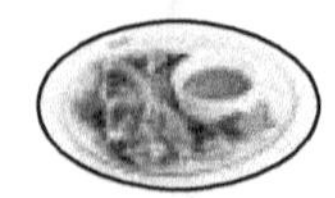 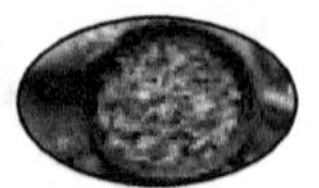

Day 18:

- **Breakfast:** Protein-Packed Egg Muffins

- **Lunch:** Broccoli and Cheese Stuffed Portobello Mushrooms

- **Dinner:** Grilled Chicken Salad

Day 19:

- **Breakfast:** Berry Bliss Yogurt Parfait

- **Lunch:** Caprese Salad

- **Dinner:** Sweet Potato and Chickpea Hash

Day 20:

- **Breakfast:** Chocolate Avocado Mousse

- **Lunch:** Mediterranean Chickpea Salad

- **Dinner:** Salmon and Asparagus Foil Pack

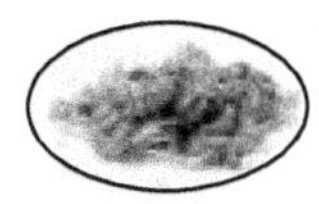 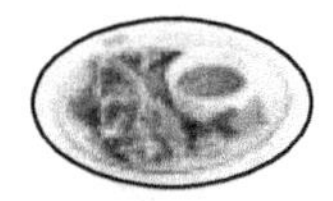 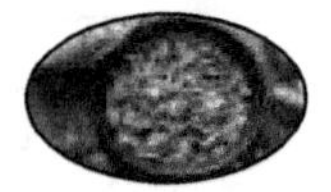

Day 21:

- **Breakfast:** Mango Coconut Chia Popsicles
- **Lunch:** Turkey Lettuce Wraps
- **Dinner:** Eggplant Parmesan

Day 22:

- **Breakfast:** Zucchini Noodles with Pesto
- **Lunch:** Cucumber and Tuna Bites
- **Dinner:** Veggie Omelette

Day 23:

- **Breakfast:** Almond Butter Banana Bites
- **Lunch:** Lentil Soup
- **Dinner:** Berry Almond Chia Pudding

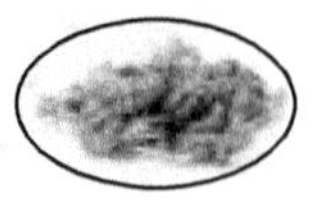 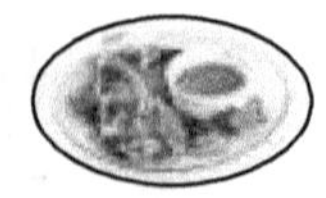 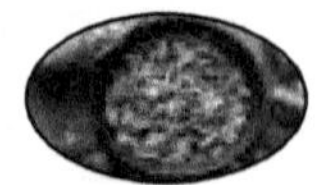

Day 24:

- **Breakfast:** Avocado and Turkey Wrap

- **Lunch:** Shrimp and Broccoli Stir-Fry

- **Dinner:** Quinoa Veggie Bowl

Day 25:

- **Breakfast:** Protein-Packed Egg Muffins

- **Lunch:** Broccoli and Cheese Stuffed Portobello Mushrooms

- **Dinner:** Grilled Chicken Salad

Day 26:

- **Breakfast:** Berry Bliss Yogurt Parfait

- **Lunch:** Caprese Salad

- **Dinner:** Sweet Potato and Chickpea Hash

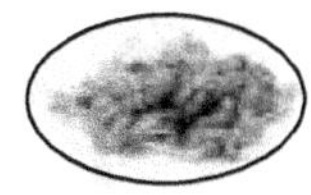 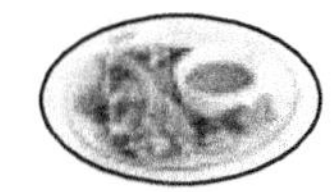 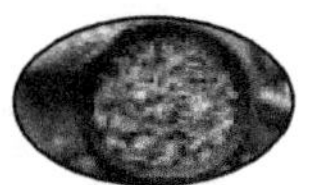

- **Breakfast:** Chocolate Avocado Mousse

- **Lunch:** Mediterranean Chickpea Salad

- **Dinner:** Salmon and Asparagus Foil Pack

- **Breakfast:** Mango Coconut Chia Popsicles

- **Lunch:** Turkey Lettuce Wraps

- **Dinner:** Eggplant Parmesan

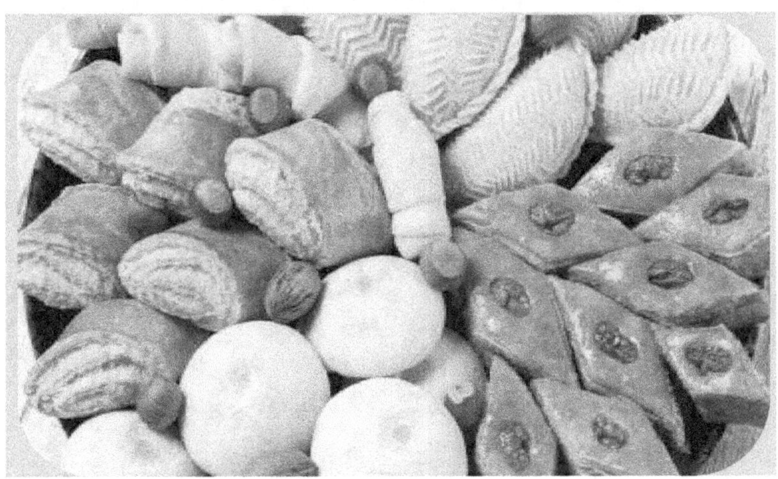

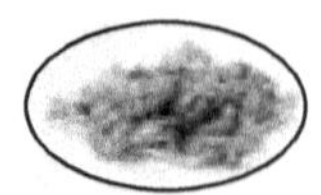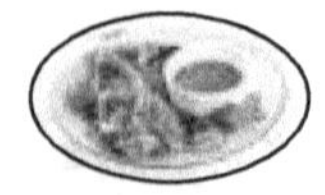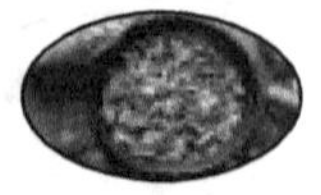

CONCLUSION

In conclusion, embarking on the journey of intermittent fasting for women over 40 offers a pathway to not only improved health but also a revitalized lifestyle. This comprehensive guide has provided a wealth of information, from understanding the science behind intermittent fasting to offering a diverse range of delicious recipes tailored to meet the unique needs of women in this age group.

As you delve into this transformative approach, remember that the key lies not only in the fasting windows but in adopting a holistic and sustainable lifestyle. Listen to your body, embrace the delicious and nutritious recipes presented in this book, and view intermittent fasting not as a restrictive practice but as a flexible and empowering tool for wellness.

The road to optimal health and well-being is a personal and evolving journey. This guide serves as a companion, offering valuable insights and practical solutions to help you navigate the–

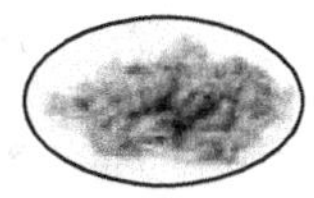 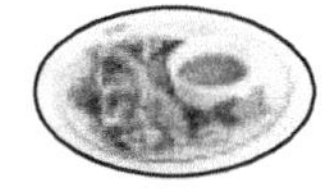 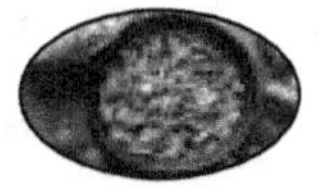

challenges and embrace the benefits of intermittent fasting. May this book empower you to make informed choices, cultivate a positive relationship with food, and embark on a fulfilling path toward a healthier, more vibrant you.

As you close the pages of this book, remember that health is a lifelong journey, and intermittent fasting is but one facet of a broader commitment to well-being. Here's to your health, happiness, and the flourishing years that lie ahead. Cheers to a life well-lived!

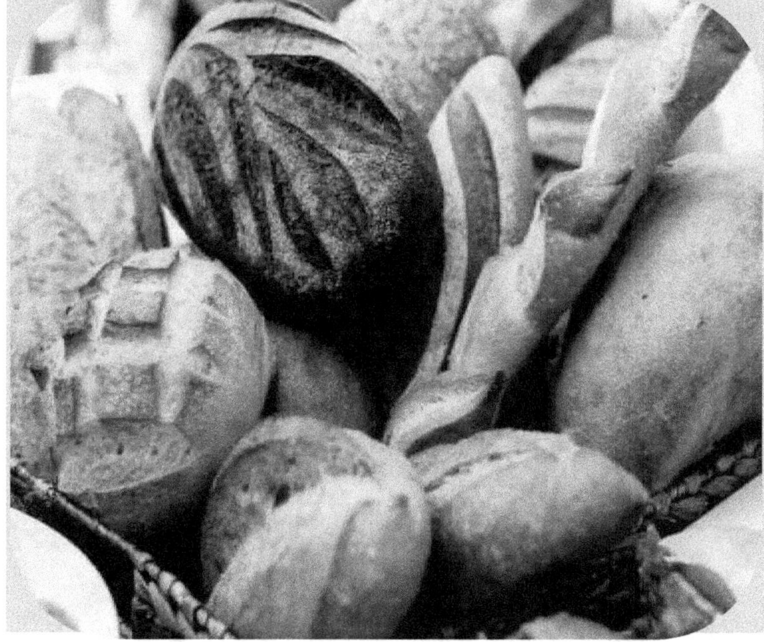

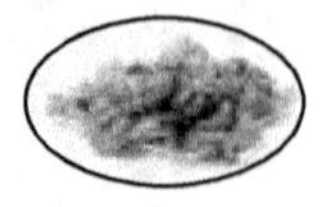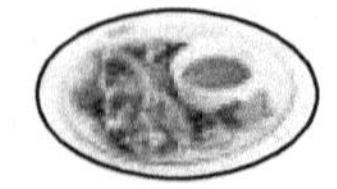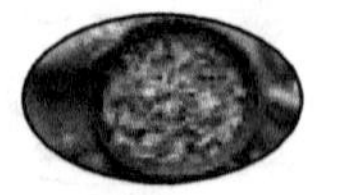

THAT'S WHY WE ARE SAYING THANK YOU…

"We know time is the unit of destiny, that's why we are saying thank you."

Dear Valued Customer,

we understand that time is a precious commodity, and we sincerely appreciate you choosing to spend a portion of it with us. Your decision to trust us with your purchase means the world to us, and we want to express our deepest gratitude.

Your support not only fuels our passion for delivering quality products but also contributes to the destiny of our business. Each customer is a vital part of our journey, and we are honored to have you

We strive to provide an exceptional shopping experience, and your satisfaction is our top priority. If you have any feedback or suggestions, we would love to hear from you. Your insights help us improve.

As a small token of our appreciation, we kindly invite you to share your experience by leaving a 5-star review. Your feedback not only boosts our morale but also assists fellow shoppers in making informed decisions.

Once again, thank you for choosing to buy this book. We look forward to serving you again and being a part of your destiny in the world of quality and excellence.

Warm regards,

Dr. Grace Hester–

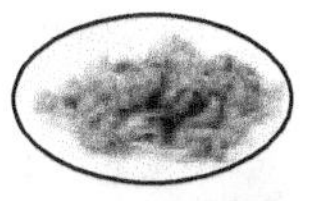
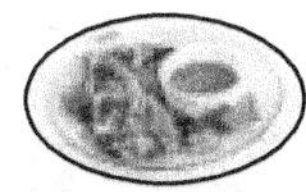
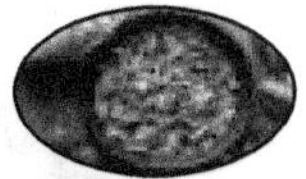

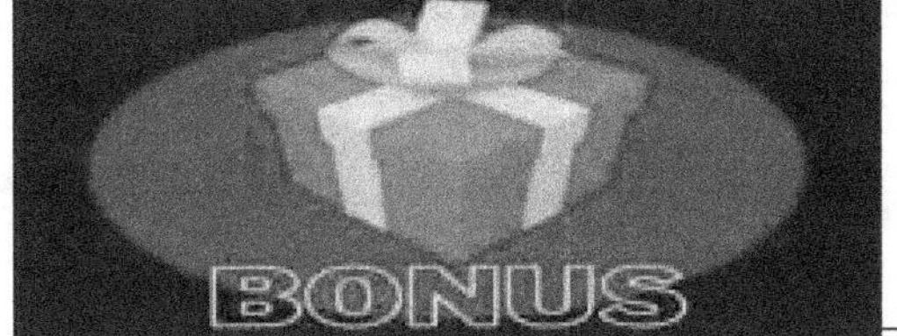

BONUS 2; 20 DAYS + MEAL PLANNER

(paperback version)

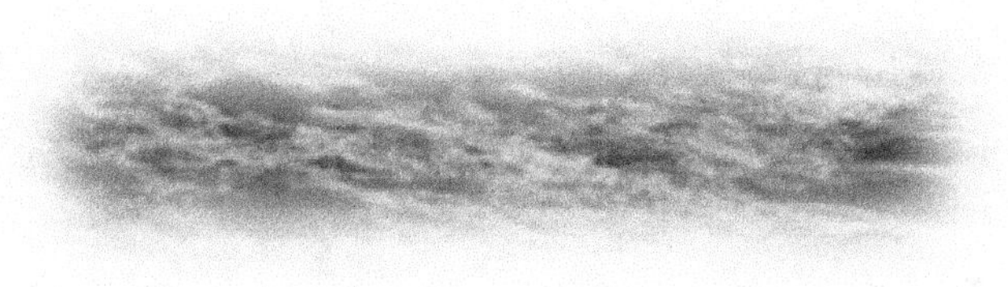

BONUS 3; SUPPORT MAIL

Gracehester.recipes@gmail.com–

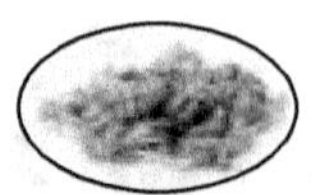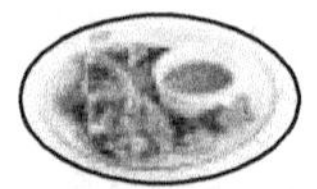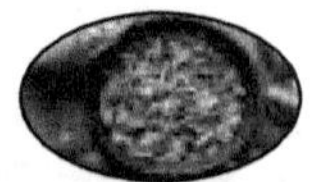

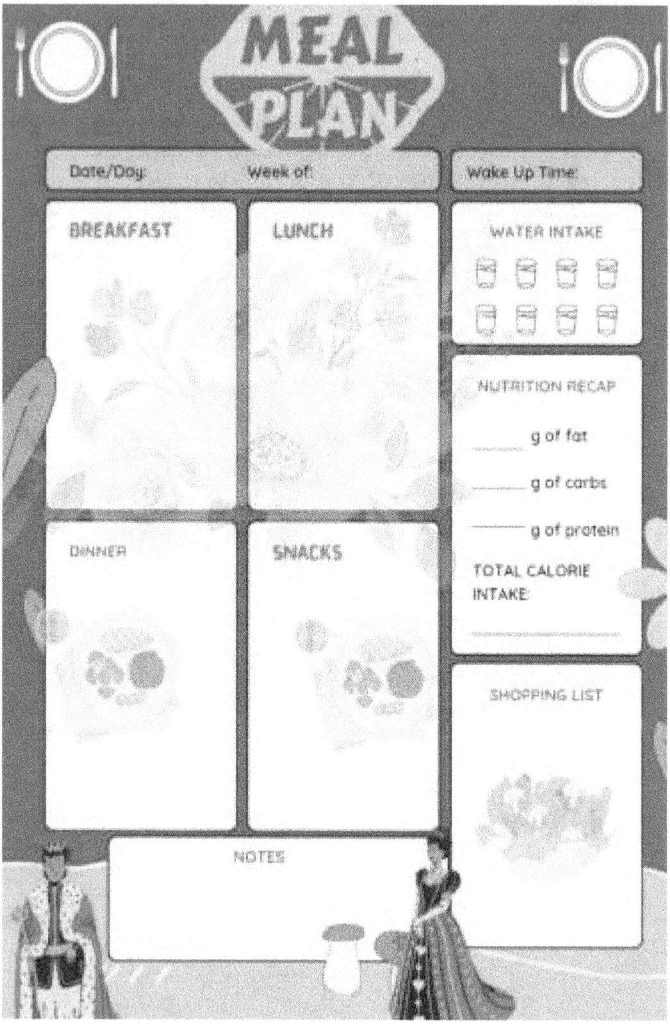

MEAL PLAN

| Date/Day: | Week of: | Wake Up Time: |

BREAKFAST

LUNCH

WATER INTAKE

NUTRITION RECAP

________ g of fat

________ g of carbs

________ g of protein

TOTAL CALORIE INTAKE:

DINNER

SNACKS

SHOPPING LIST

NOTES

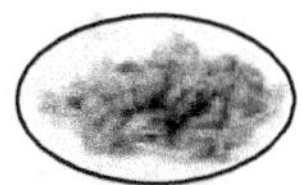 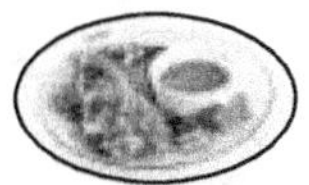 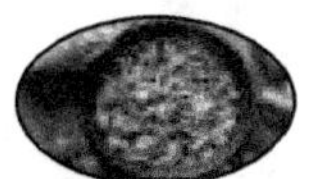

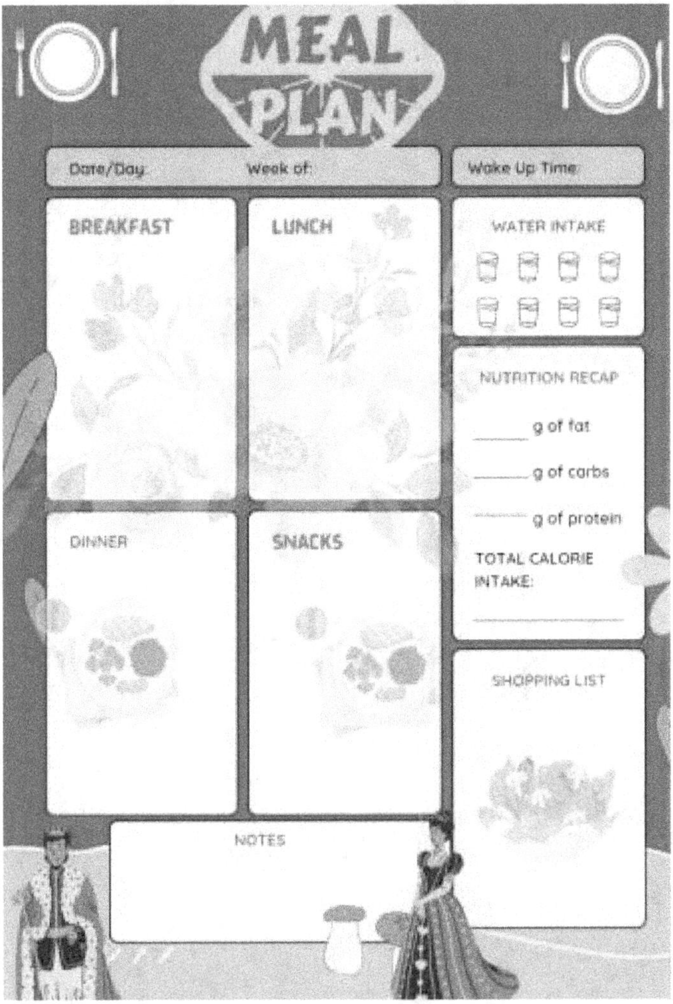

MEAL PLAN

| Date/Day: | Week of: | Wake Up Time: |

BREAKFAST

LUNCH

WATER INTAKE

NUTRITION RECAP

_________ g of fat

_________ g of carbs

_________ g of protein

TOTAL CALORIE INTAKE:

____

DINNER

SNACKS

SHOPPING LIST

NOTES

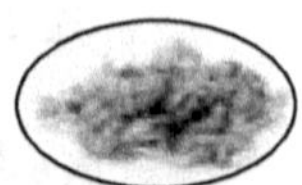 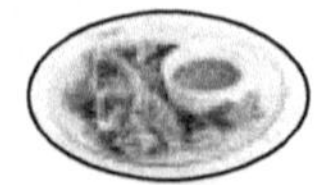 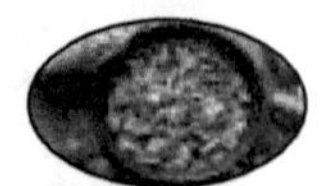

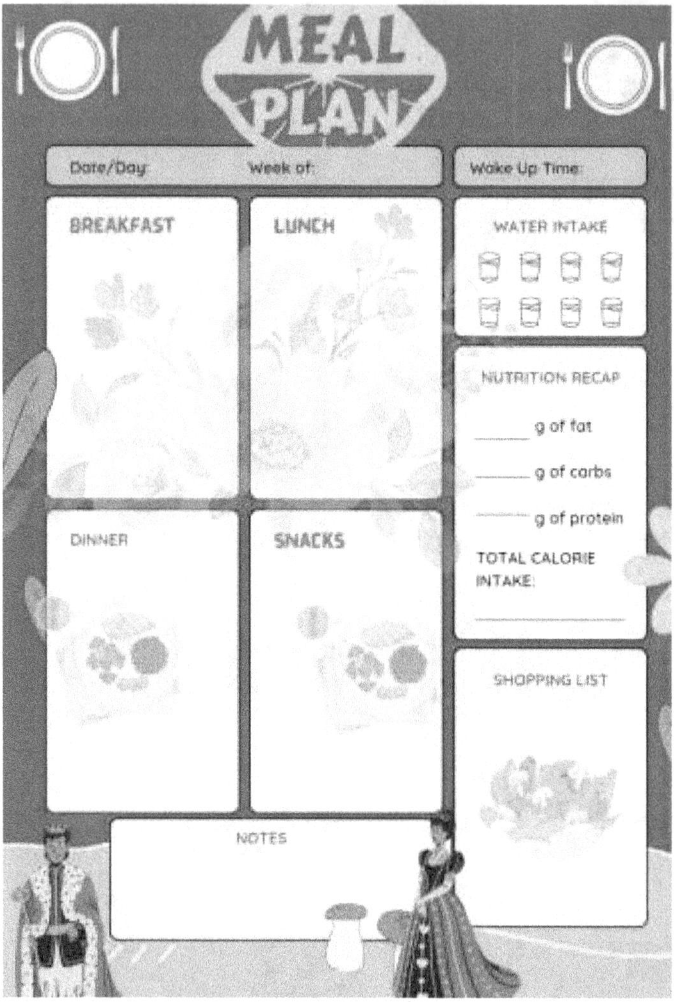

MEAL PLAN

Date/Day:	Week of:	Wake Up Time:

BREAKFAST

LUNCH

WATER INTAKE

NUTRITION RECAP

__________ g of fat

__________ g of carbs

__________ g of protein

TOTAL CALORIE INTAKE:

____

DINNER

SNACKS

SHOPPING LIST

NOTES

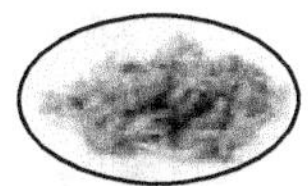 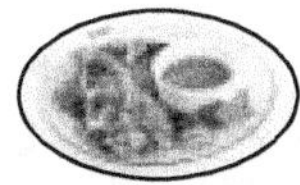 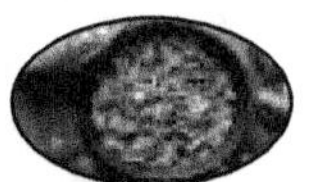

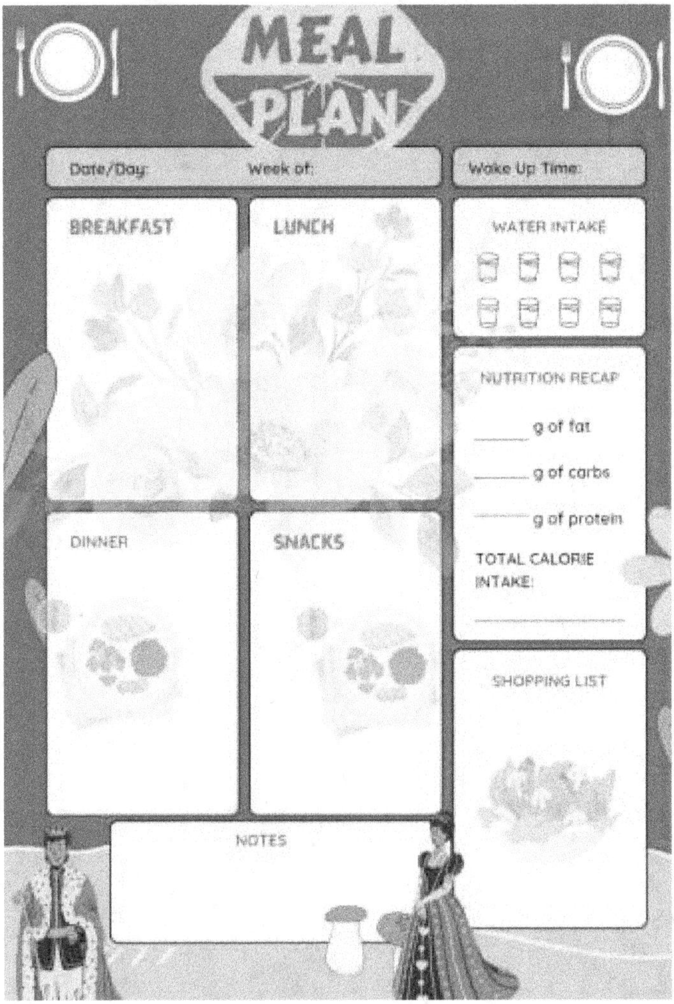

MEAL PLAN

| Date/Day: | Week of: | Woke Up Time: |

BREAKFAST

LUNCH

WATER INTAKE

NUTRITION RECAP

__________ g of fat

__________ g of carbs

__________ g of protein

TOTAL CALORIE INTAKE:

DINNER

SNACKS

SHOPPING LIST

NOTES

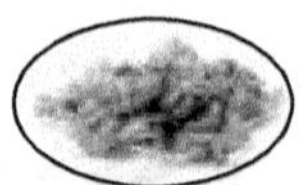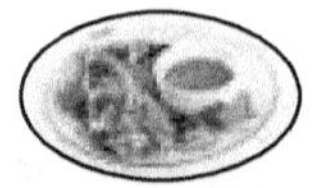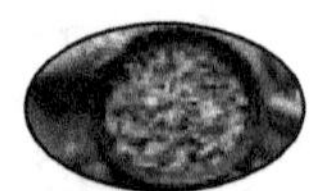

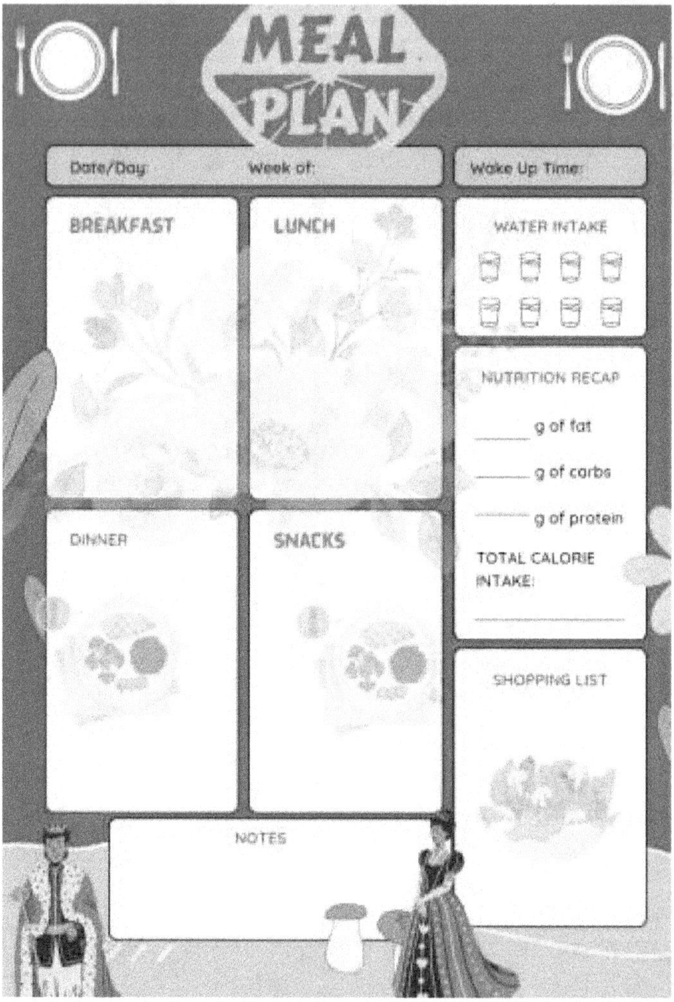

MEAL PLAN

| Date/Day: | Week of: | Wake Up Time: |

BREAKFAST

LUNCH

WATER INTAKE

NUTRITION RECAP

_______ g of fat

_______ g of carbs

_______ g of protein

TOTAL CALORIE INTAKE:

____

DINNER

SNACKS

SHOPPING LIST

NOTES

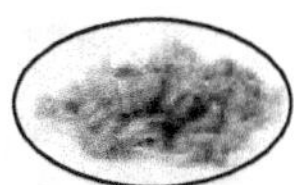 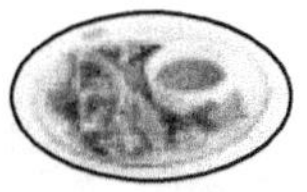 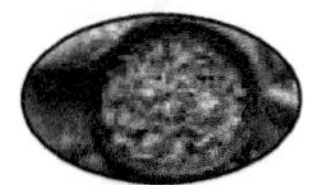

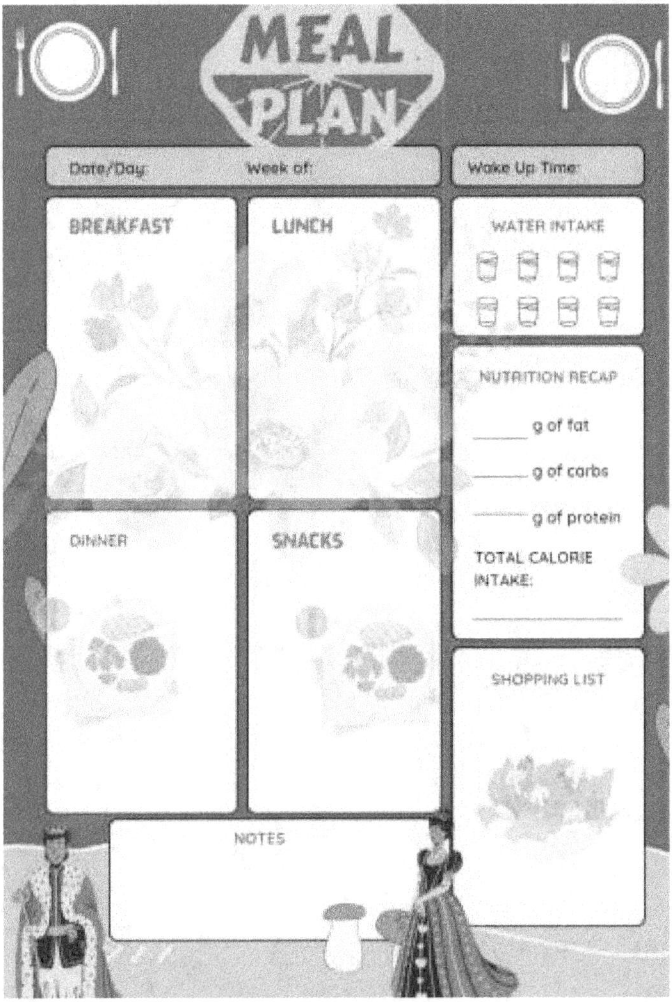

MEAL PLAN

| Date/Day | Week of: | Wake Up Time: |

BREAKFAST

LUNCH

WATER INTAKE

NUTRITION RECAP

__________ g of fat

__________ g of carbs

__________ g of protein

TOTAL CALORIE INTAKE:

____

DINNER

SNACKS

SHOPPING LIST

NOTES

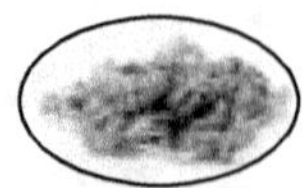

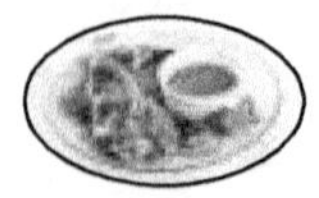

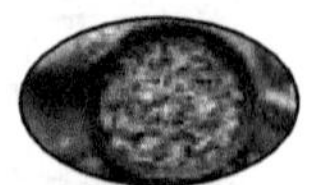

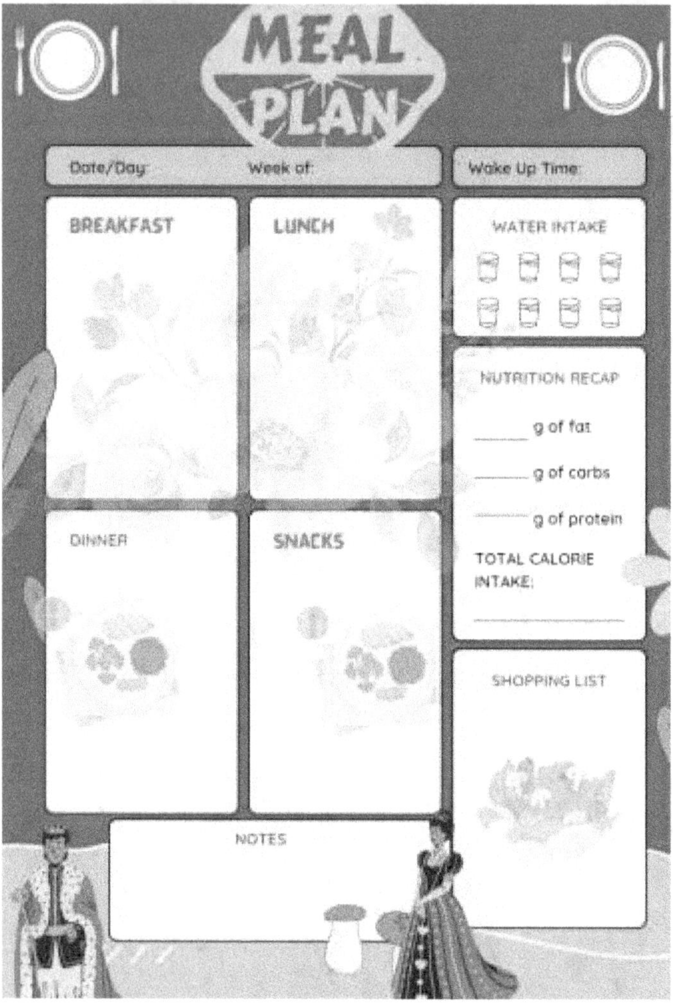

MEAL PLAN
Date/Day:
Week of:
Wake Up Time:
BREAKFAST
LUNCH
WATER INTAKE
NUTRITION RECAP
g of fat
g of carbs
g of protein
TOTAL CALORIE INTAKE:
DINNER
SNACKS
SHOPPING LIST
NOTES

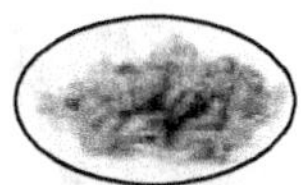 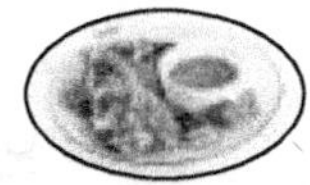 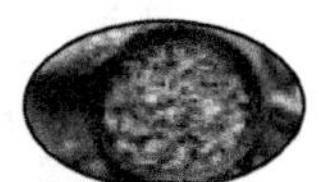

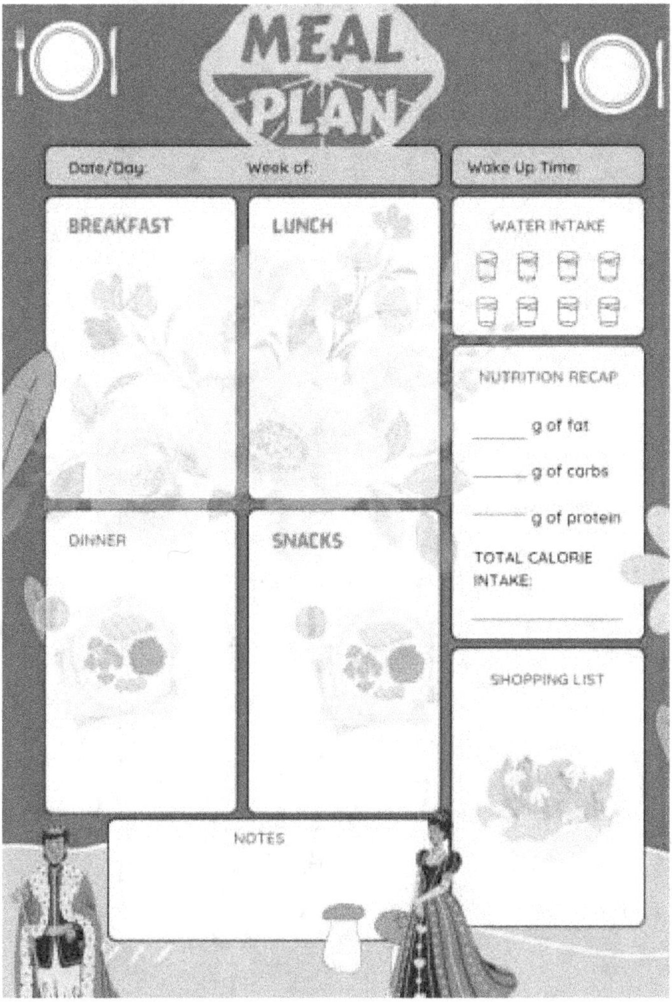

MEAL PLAN

| Date/Day: | Week of: | Wake Up Time: |

BREAKFAST

LUNCH

WATER INTAKE

NUTRITION RECAP

__________ g of fat

__________ g of carbs

__________ g of protein

TOTAL CALORIE INTAKE:

____

DINNER

SNACKS

SHOPPING LIST

NOTES

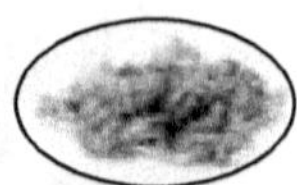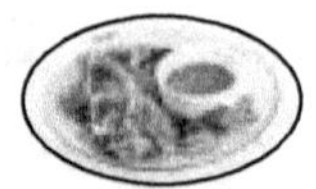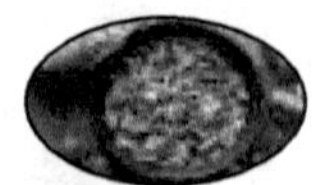

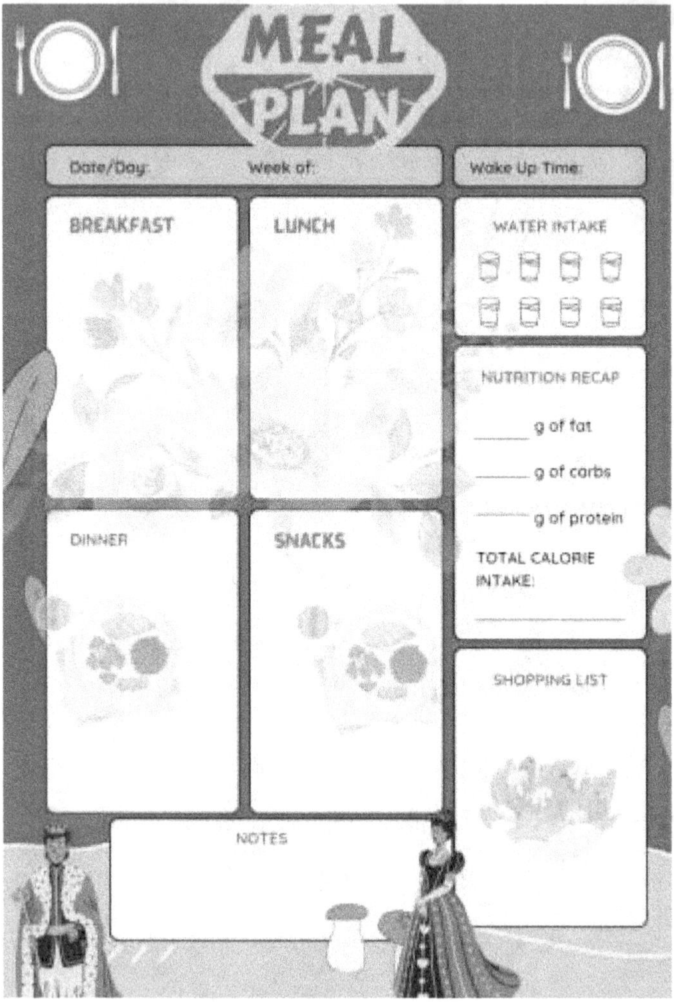

MEAL PLAN

| Date/Day: | Week of: | Wake Up Time: |

BREAKFAST

LUNCH

WATER INTAKE

NUTRITION RECAP

_______ g of fat

_______ g of carbs

_______ g of protein

TOTAL CALORIE INTAKE:

____

DINNER

SNACKS

SHOPPING LIST

NOTES

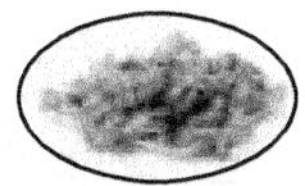 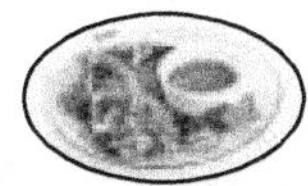 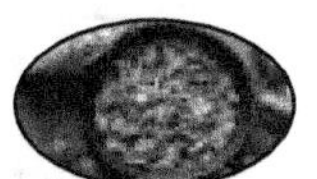

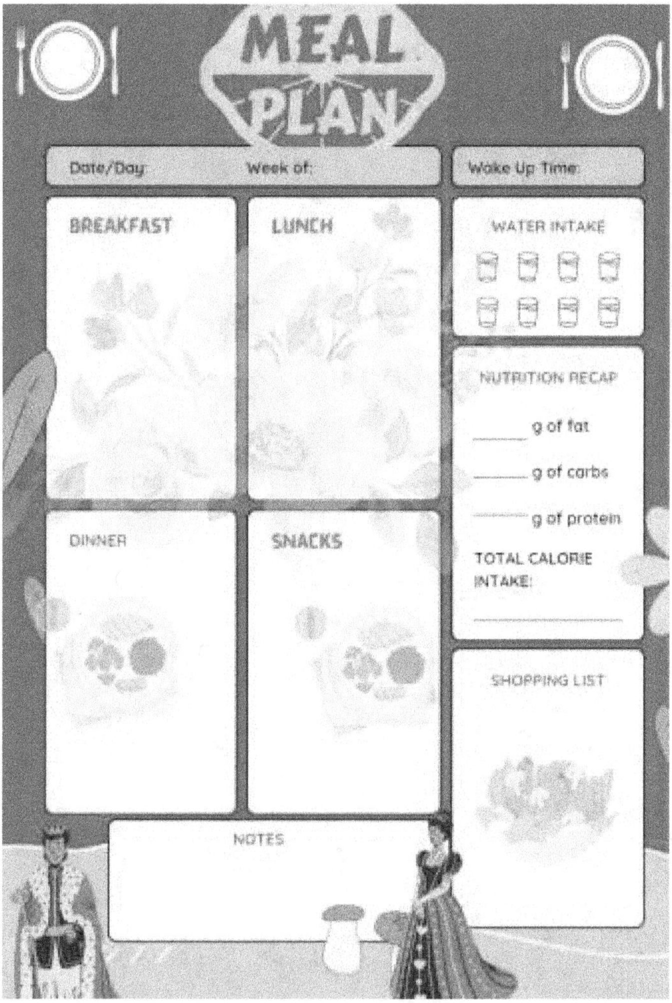

MEAL PLAN

Date/Day:	Week of:	Woke Up Time:

BREAKFAST

LUNCH

WATER INTAKE

NUTRITION RECAP

______ g of fat

______ g of carbs

______ g of protein

TOTAL CALORIE INTAKE:

____

DINNER

SNACKS

SHOPPING LIST

NOTES

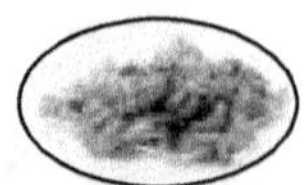
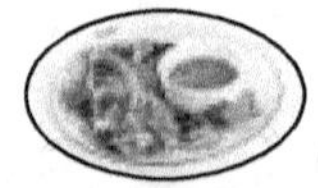
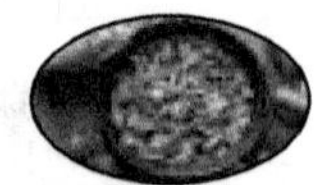

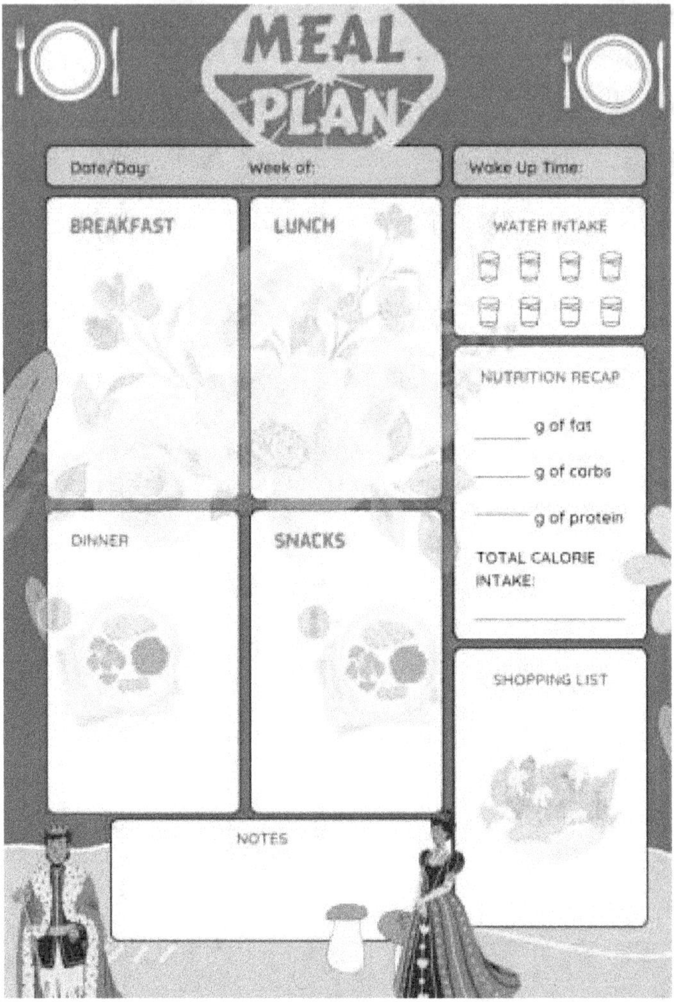

MEAL PLAN

| Date/Day: | Week of: | Wake Up Time: |

BREAKFAST

LUNCH

WATER INTAKE

NUTRITION RECAP

_______ g of fat

_______ g of carbs

_______ g of protein

TOTAL CALORIE INTAKE:

____

DINNER

SNACKS

SHOPPING LIST

NOTES

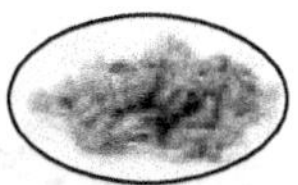 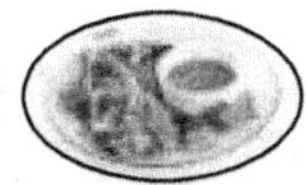 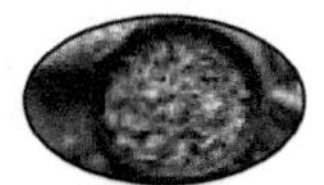

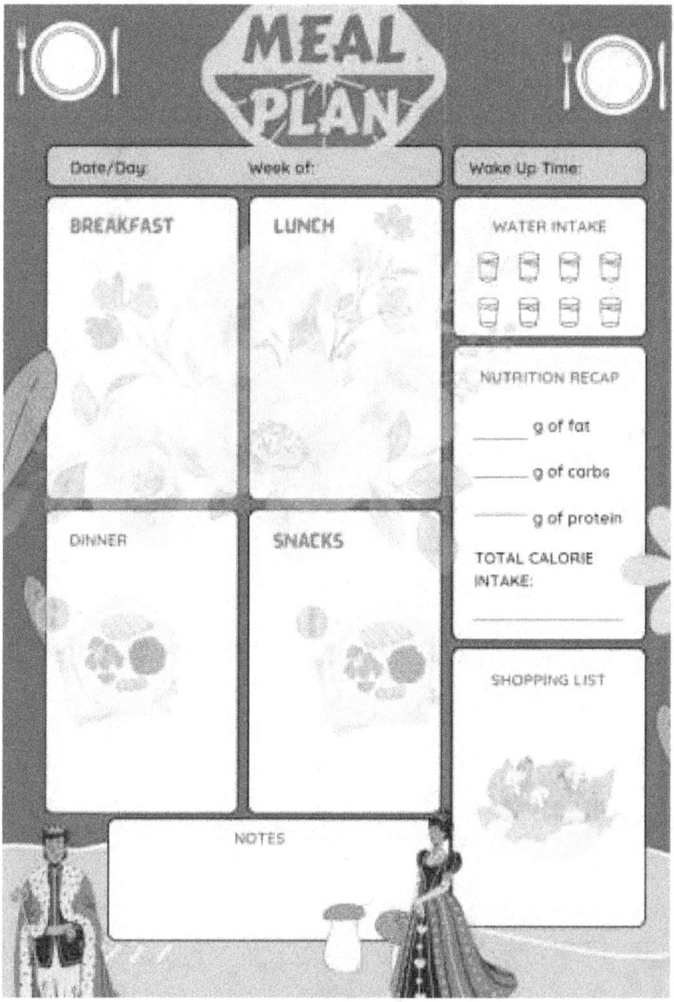

MEAL PLAN

| Date/Day: | Week of: | Wake Up Time: |

BREAKFAST

LUNCH

WATER INTAKE

NUTRITION RECAP

_______ g of fat

_______ g of carbs

_______ g of protein

TOTAL CALORIE INTAKE:

____

DINNER

SNACKS

SHOPPING LIST

NOTES

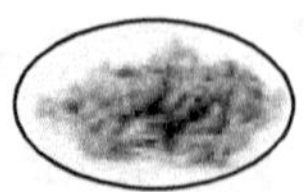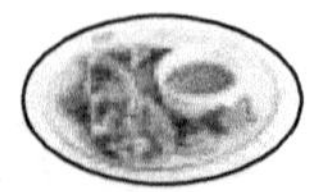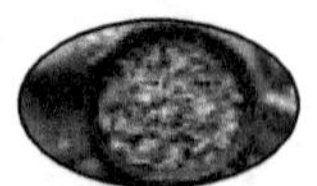

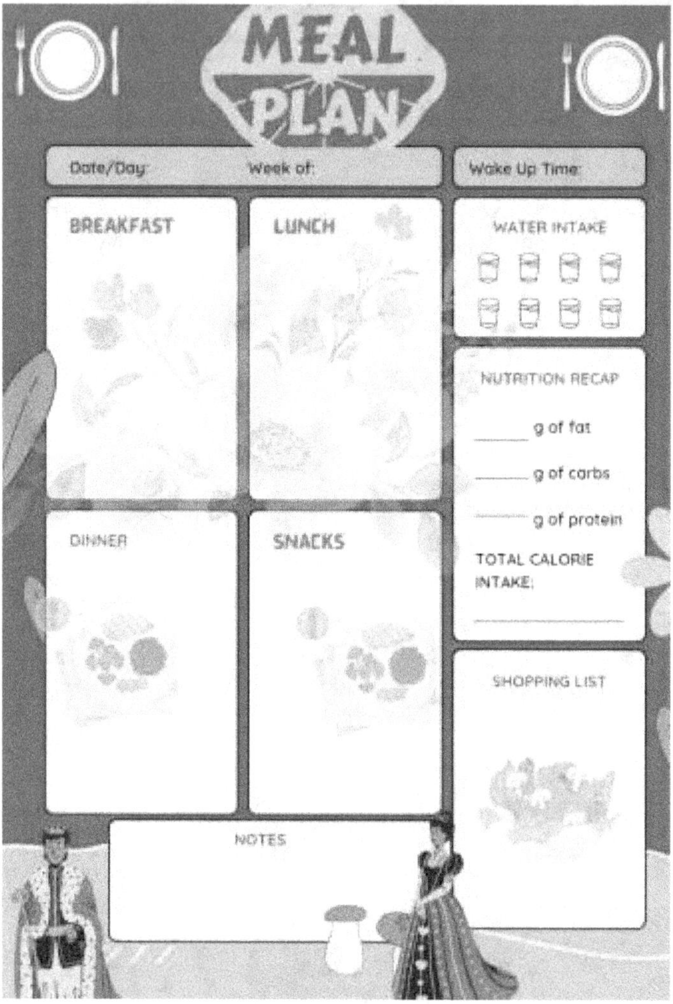

MEAL PLAN

| Date/Day: | Week of: | Wake Up Time: |

BREAKFAST

LUNCH

WATER INTAKE

NUTRITION RECAP

_______ g of fat

_______ g of carbs

_______ g of protein

TOTAL CALORIE INTAKE:

____

DINNER

SNACKS

SHOPPING LIST

NOTES

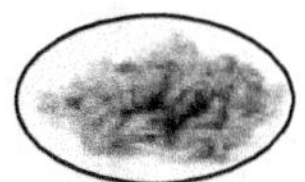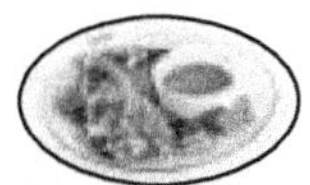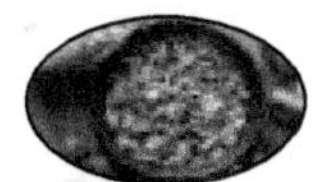

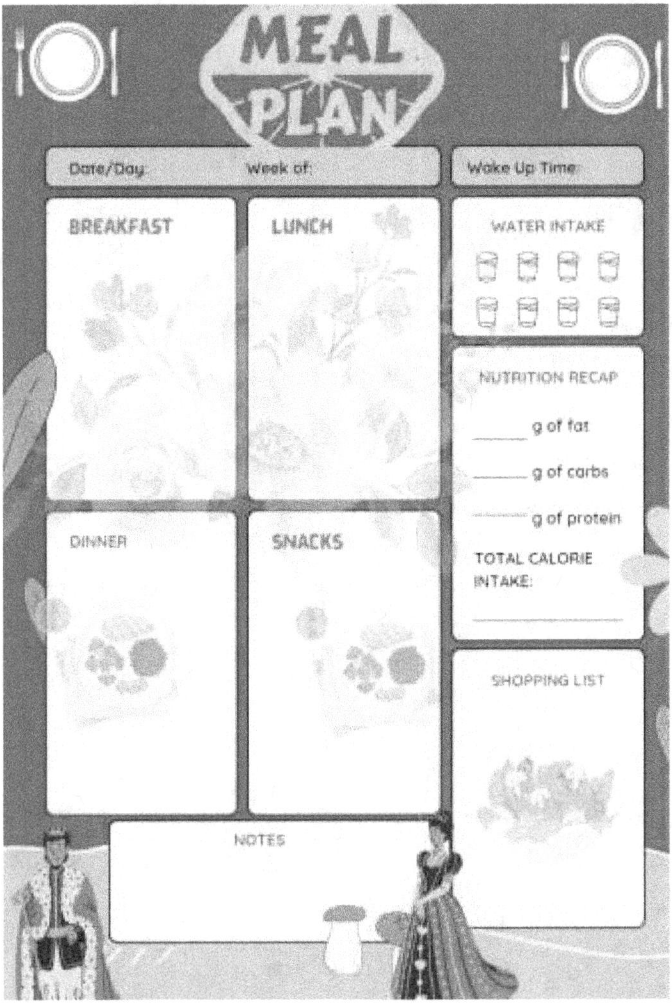

MEAL PLAN

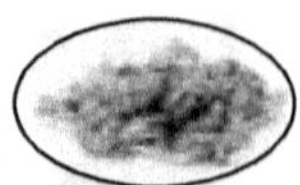
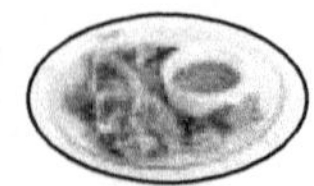
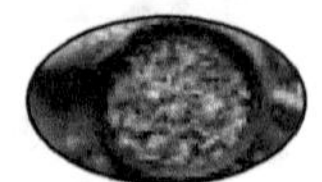

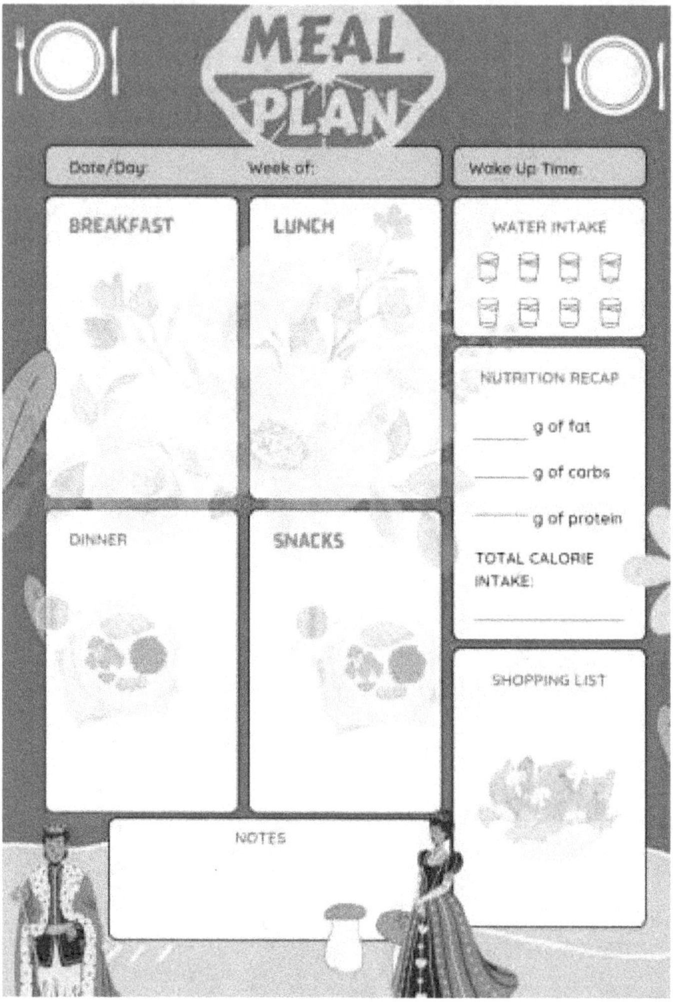

MEAL PLAN

| Date/Day: | Week of: | Wake Up Time: |

BREAKFAST

LUNCH

WATER INTAKE

NUTRITION RECAP

_______ g of fat

_______ g of carbs

_______ g of protein

TOTAL CALORIE INTAKE:

____

DINNER

SNACKS

SHOPPING LIST

NOTES

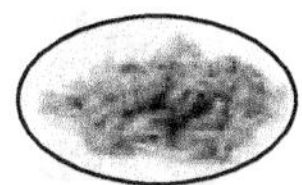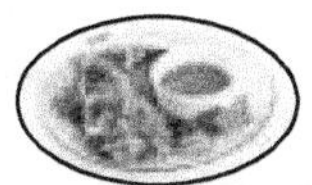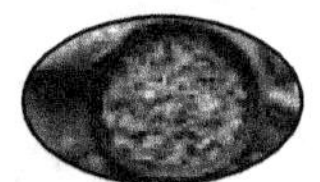

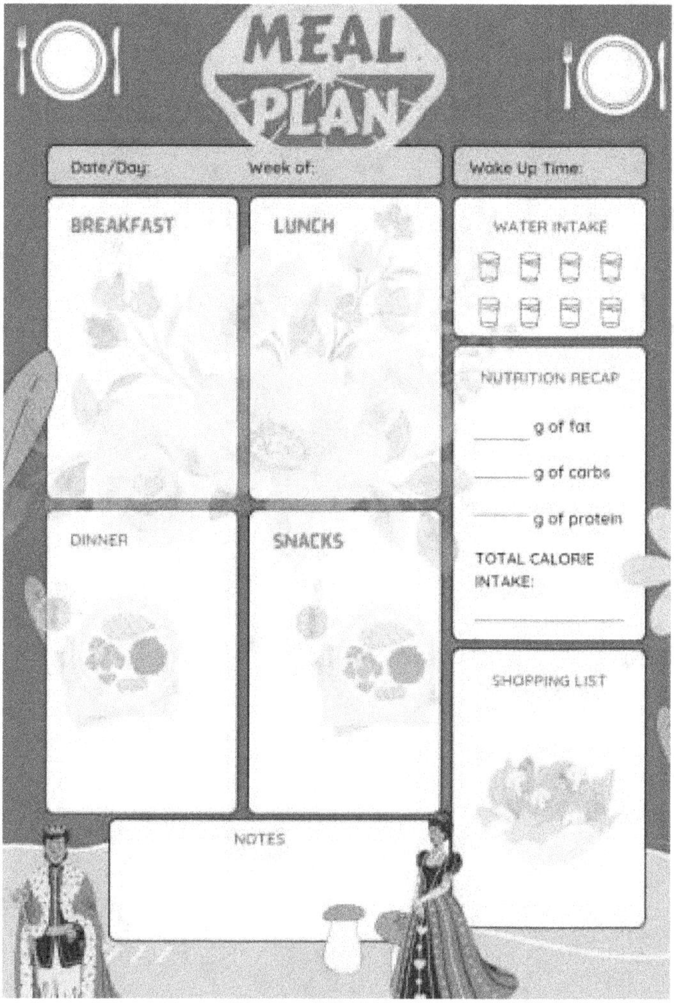

MEAL PLAN

Date/Day:	Week of:	Woke Up Time:

BREAKFAST

LUNCH

WATER INTAKE

NUTRITION RECAP

__________ g of fat

__________ g of carbs

__________ g of protein

TOTAL CALORIE INTAKE:

____

DINNER

SNACKS

SHOPPING LIST

NOTES

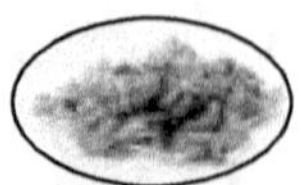 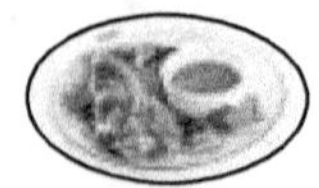 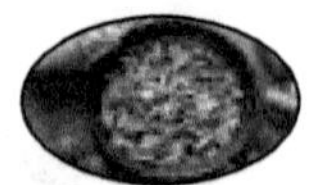

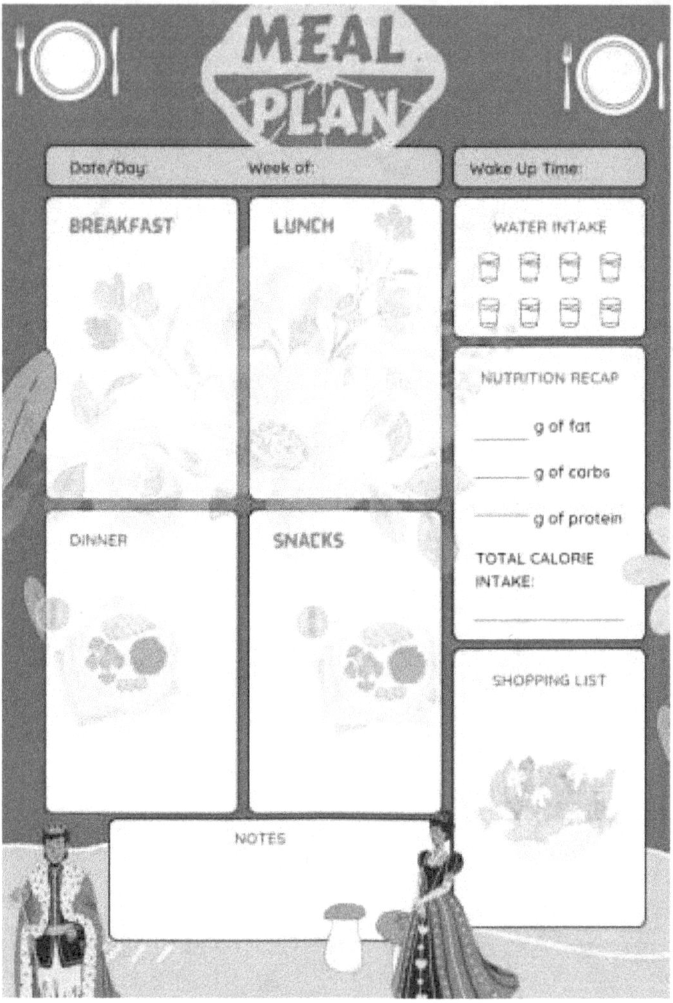

MEAL PLAN

| Date/Day: | Week of: | Wake Up Time: |

BREAKFAST

LUNCH

WATER INTAKE

NUTRITION RECAP

_________ g of fat

_________ g of carbs

_________ g of protein

TOTAL CALORIE INTAKE:

____

DINNER

SNACKS

SHOPPING LIST

NOTES

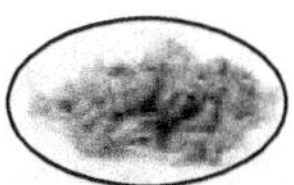 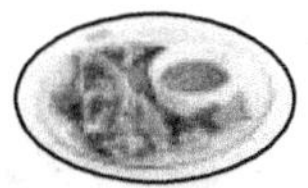 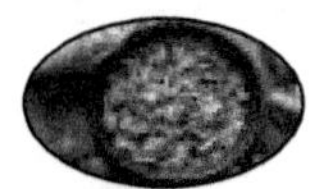

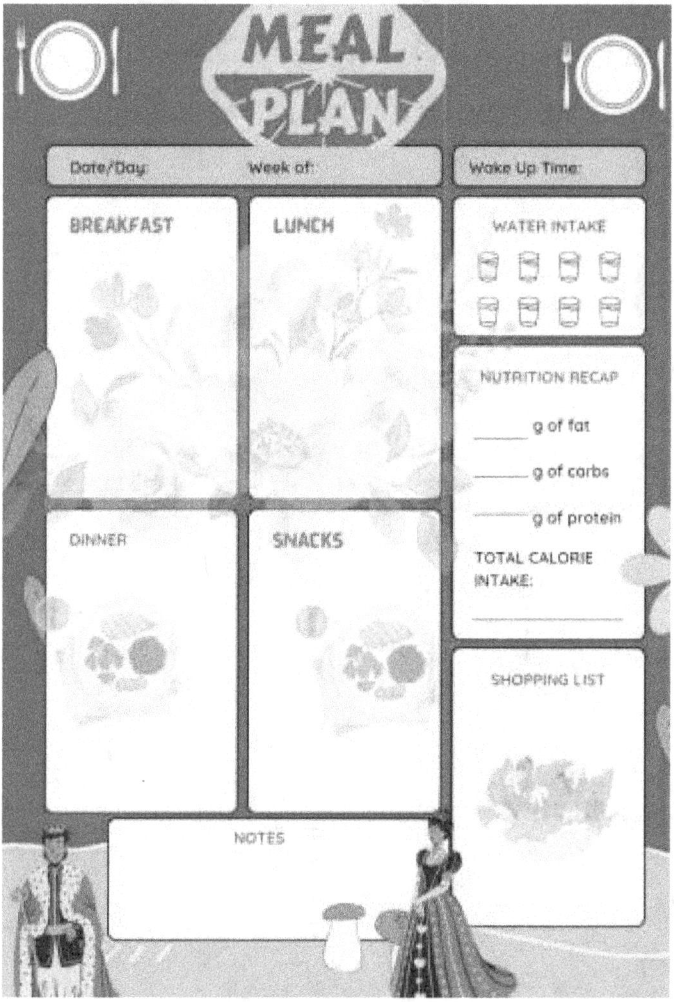

MEAL PLAN

| Date/Day: | Week of: | Wake Up Time: |

BREAKFAST

LUNCH

WATER INTAKE

NUTRITION RECAP

_______ g of fat

_______ g of carbs

_______ g of protein

TOTAL CALORIE INTAKE:

____

DINNER

SNACKS

SHOPPING LIST

NOTES

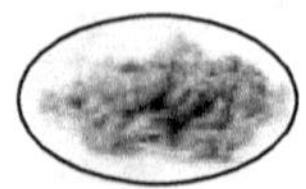 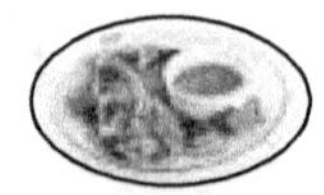 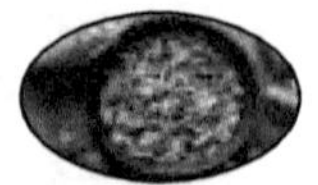

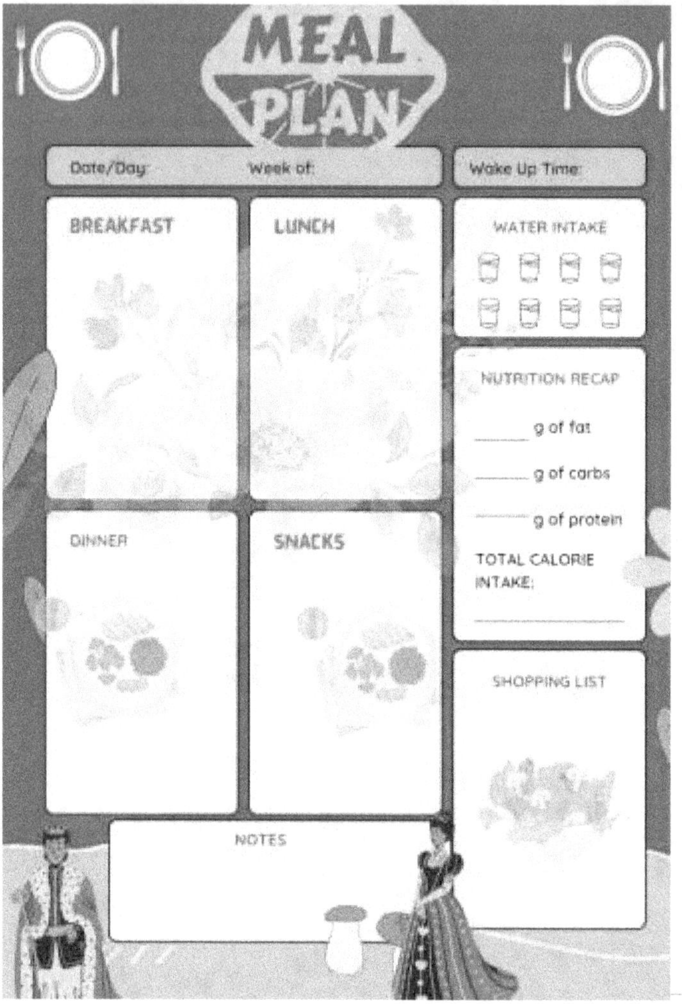

MEAL PLAN

| Date/Day: | Week of: | Wake Up Time: |

BREAKFAST

LUNCH

WATER INTAKE

NUTRITION RECAP

________ g of fat

________ g of carbs

________ g of protein

TOTAL CALORIE INTAKE:

____

DINNER

SNACKS

SHOPPING LIST

NOTES

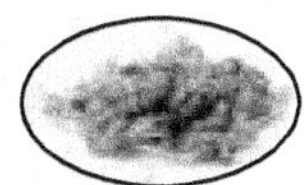 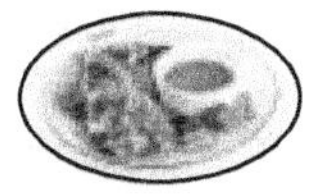 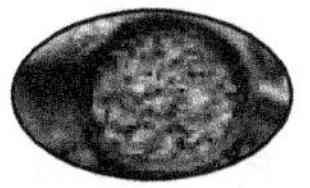

We are sure you enjoyed reading this straight to the point book, to get more on Dr. Grace Hester, scan the QR code below;

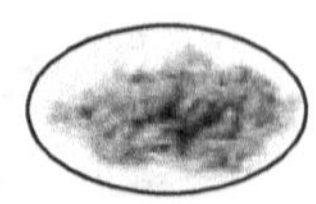 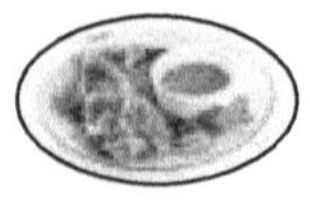 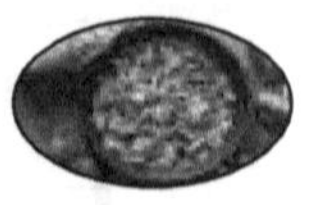